THE GUIDE TO

LESBIAN SEX

JUDE SCHELL

Hylas Publishing®
129 Main Street, Suite C
Irvington, NY 10533
www.hylaspublishing.com

Hylas Publishing
Publisher: Sean Moore
Creative Director: Karen Prince
Art Directors: Gus Yoo, Edwin Kuo
Editorial Director: Gail Greiner
Production Managers: Sarah Reilly, Wayne Ellis

Project Credits
Designer: Marian Purcell
Photoshop: Mikhaylovich Smith
Editor: Gail Greiner
Photographer: Robert Wright
Proofreader: Solange Xanadu

ISBN: 1-59258-137-4

Library of Congress Cataloging-in-Publication Data available upon request.
Distributed in the United States by National Book Network
Distributed in Canada by Kate Walker & Company, Ltd.
First American Edition published in 2005
10 9 8 7 6 5 4 3 2 1

THE GUIDE TO
LESBIAN SEX

JUDE SCHELL

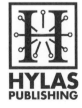

HYLAS
PUBLISHING

for Aimée,
my partner in life and love

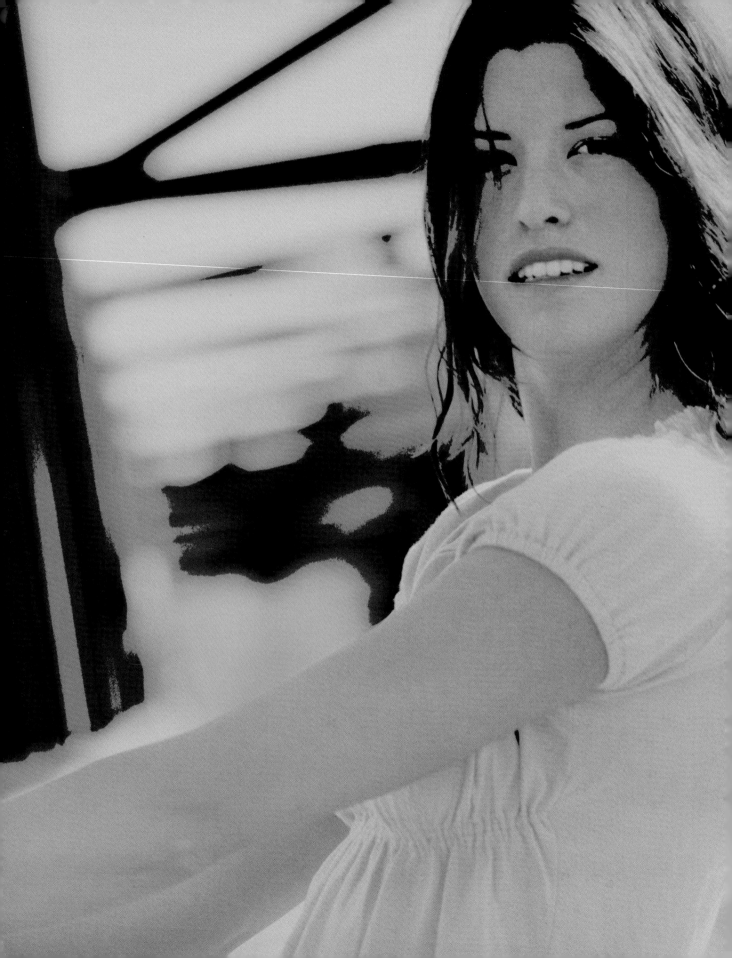

contents

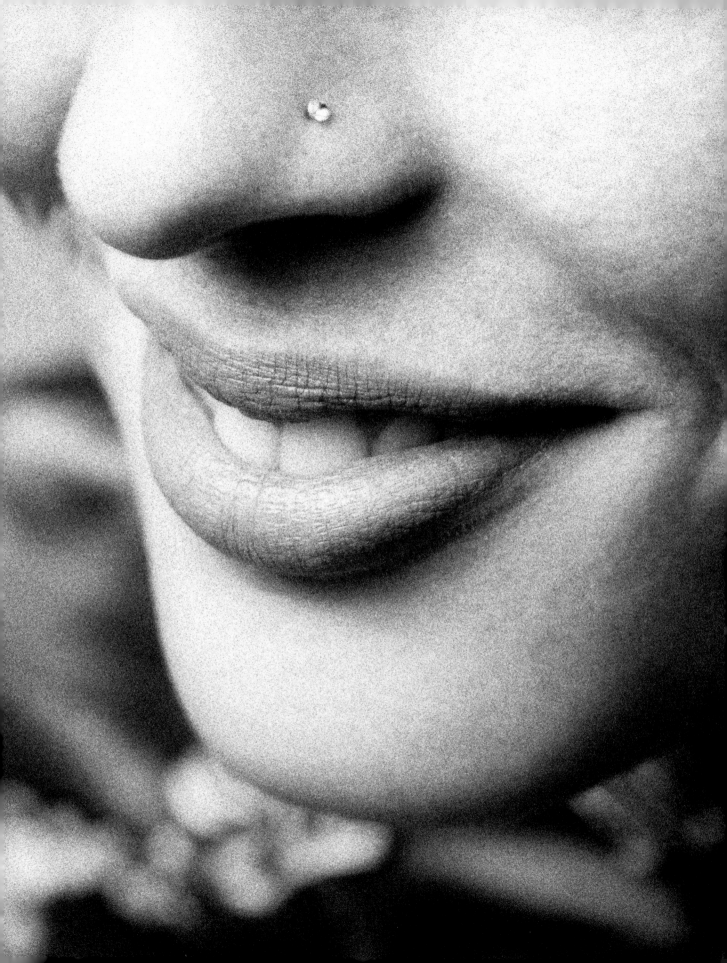

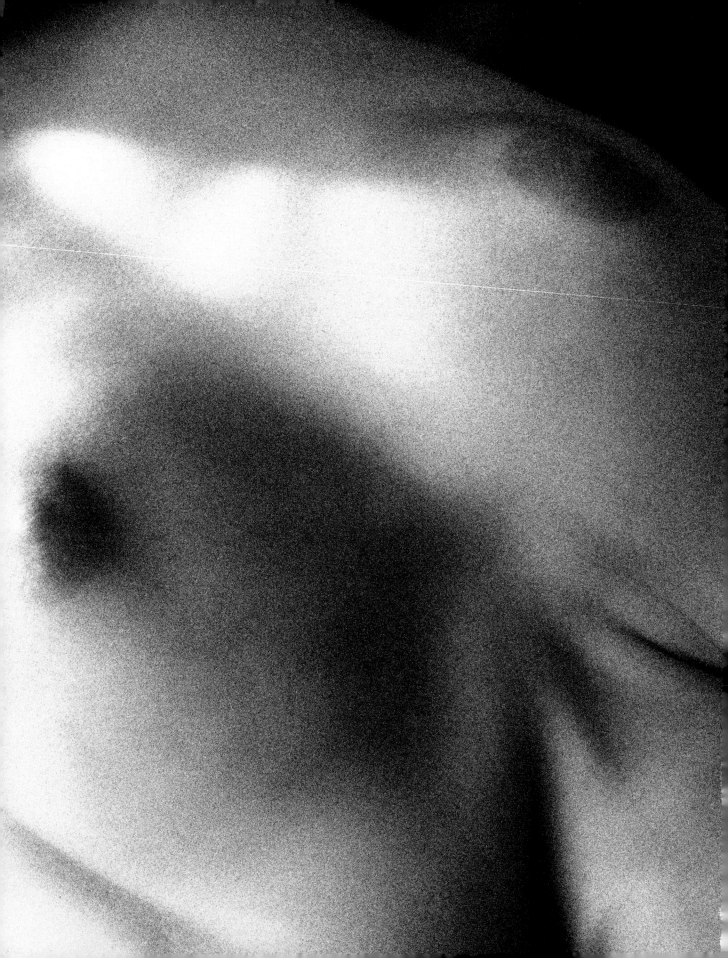

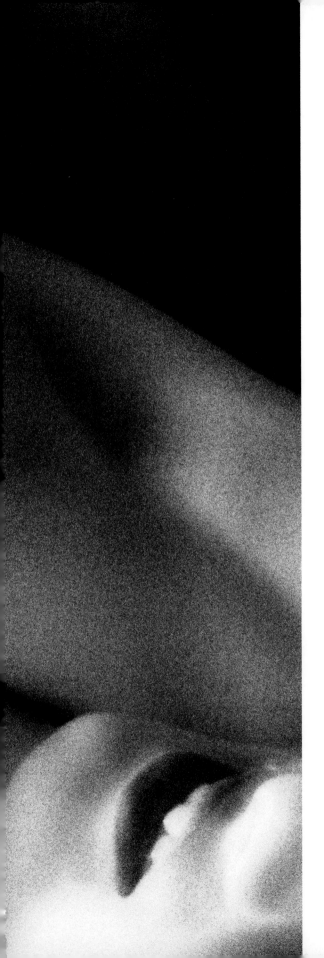

introduction

We are by nature sexual beings, yet sexuality is frequently the most suppressed and least explored element of a woman's character. Balance is the key to a happy and healthy life, so it is vital that we nurture our sexuality. When we allow the sensual, emotional, spiritual, and intellectual facets of our lives to be addressed equally, it is possible for them to co-exist harmoniously, enabling us to pursue and achieve the fulfilling life we imagine.

When we embrace our sexuality with confidence, we can anticipate, actively seek, and experience truly great sex. Women are highly sophisticated, curious, and passionate. The desires that drive us to seduce and be seduced are dynamic and often surprising. If we take on the exhilarating challenge of deconstructing our desire, an array of possibilities is revealed to us. *The Guide to Lesbian Sex* encourages and is designed to facilitate a deeper exploration of desire and other essential aspects of our sexuality.

The female body is intended to give and receive pleasure. The clitoris, a woman's major pleasure center, exists for no other purpose than for our sexual enjoyment. By learning about our erogenous zones like the clitoris, nipples, and lips, a woman can unveil and develop her own sexual proclivities. We can flirt, nibble, and be naughty to reenergize our sex lives, rediscover the pleasure in taste and touch to intensify a delicious foreplay session. We can enhance our lesbian lovemaking skills by pondering the joys of adept fingers and the sensuality of wetness. In doing this we allow ourselves and our lovers the opportunity to reach new heights of sexual satisfaction.

A book about two women making love is possible because of the inspiring visionaries, revolutionaries, and others who fight to liberate women. We continue to reinforce their groundwork to reach higher levels of tolerance, equality, and ultimately the acceptance and celebration of all people, regardless of where we place ourselves on the bell curve of sexual preference, identity, and experience.

I invite you to read *The Guide to Lesbian Sex* if you are gay, straight, bisexual, transgender, a man or a woman, alone or with a friend. Come as you are, come what may, come together and come often. Allow the blend of social psychology, physiology, ponderings, and erotica to incite your imagination and inspire the exploration of all that is possible between two women.

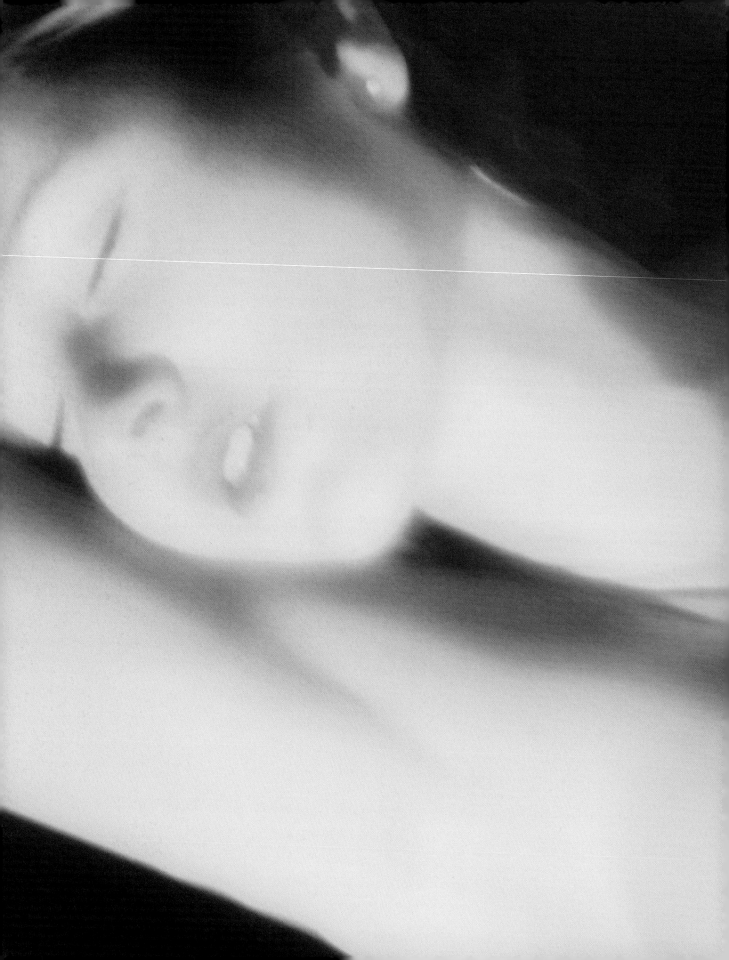

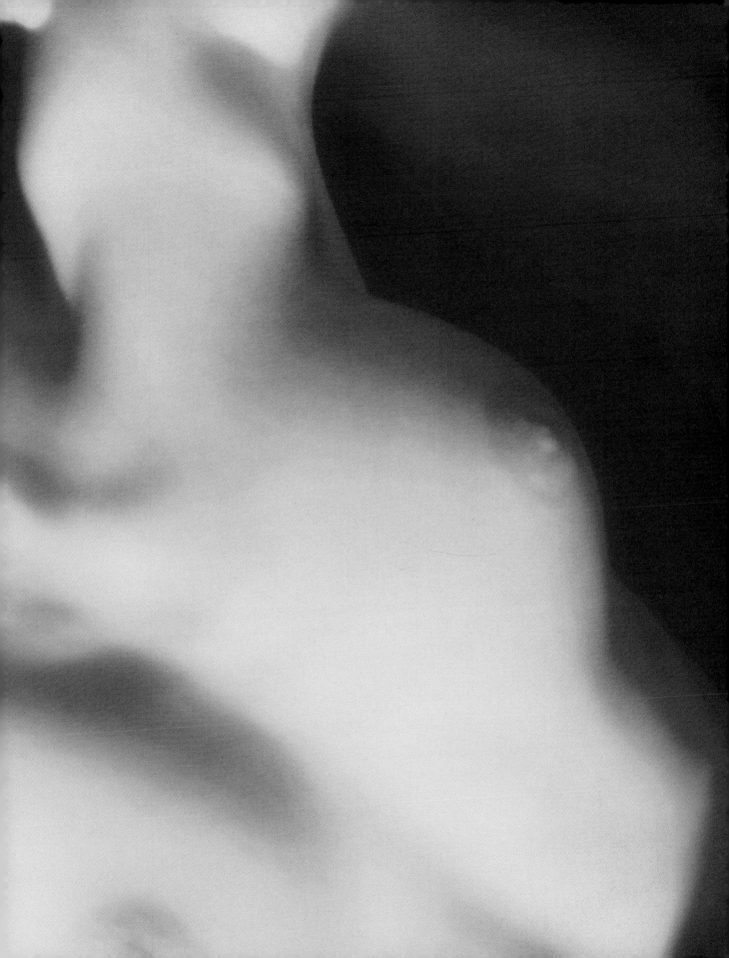

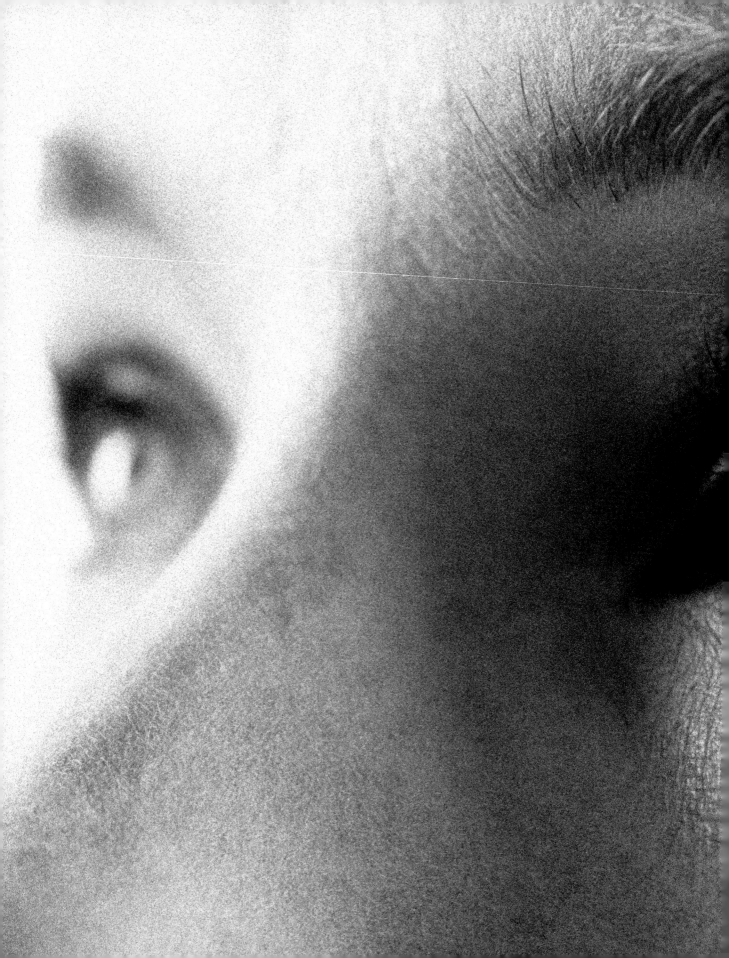

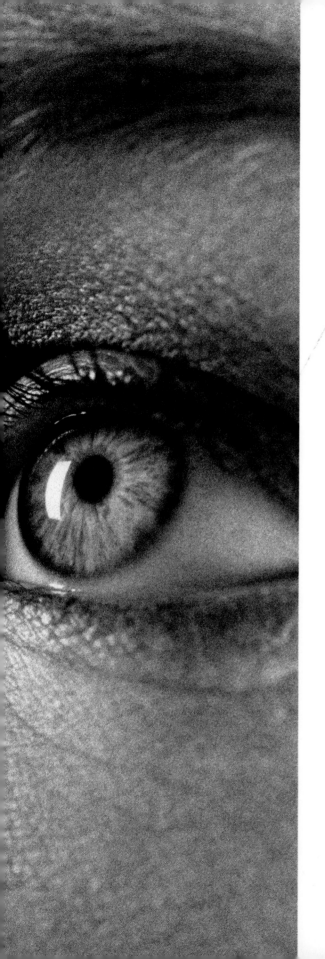

We all wish for something. Often what we wish for is tangible; we want to possess the object of our desire—whatever it may be—to fulfill a physical, sensual, intellectual, or emotional need. Other yearnings are less tangible, such as spiritual enlightenment, world peace, or true love. At its most complicated and powerful, desire is an emotion rooted in passion, and it is passion that drives our most fulfilling pursuits, including the pursuits of sex and love.

desire

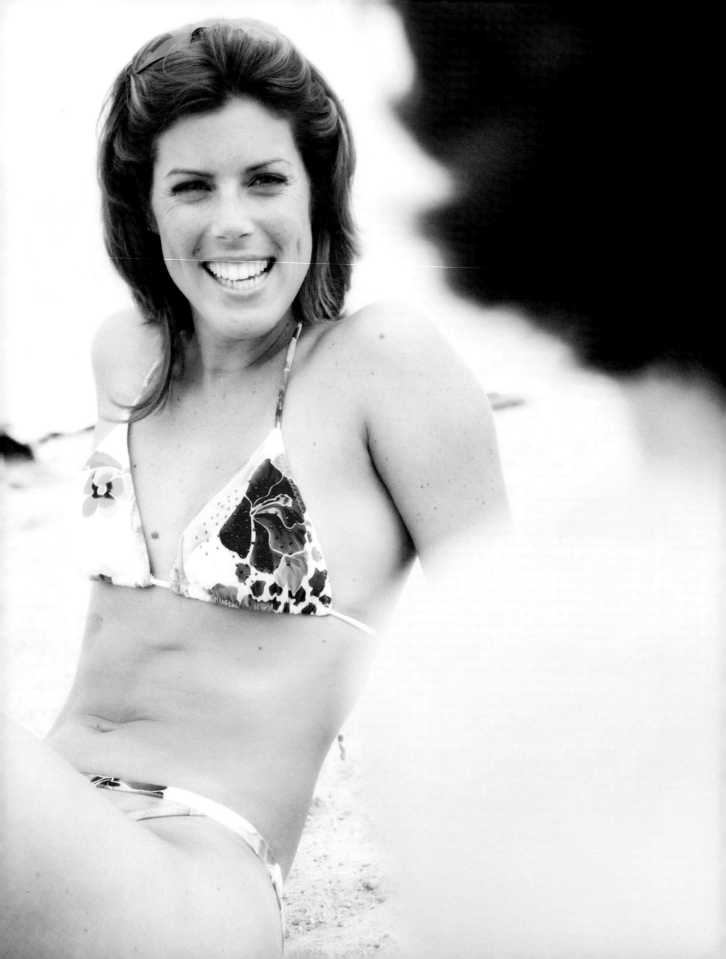

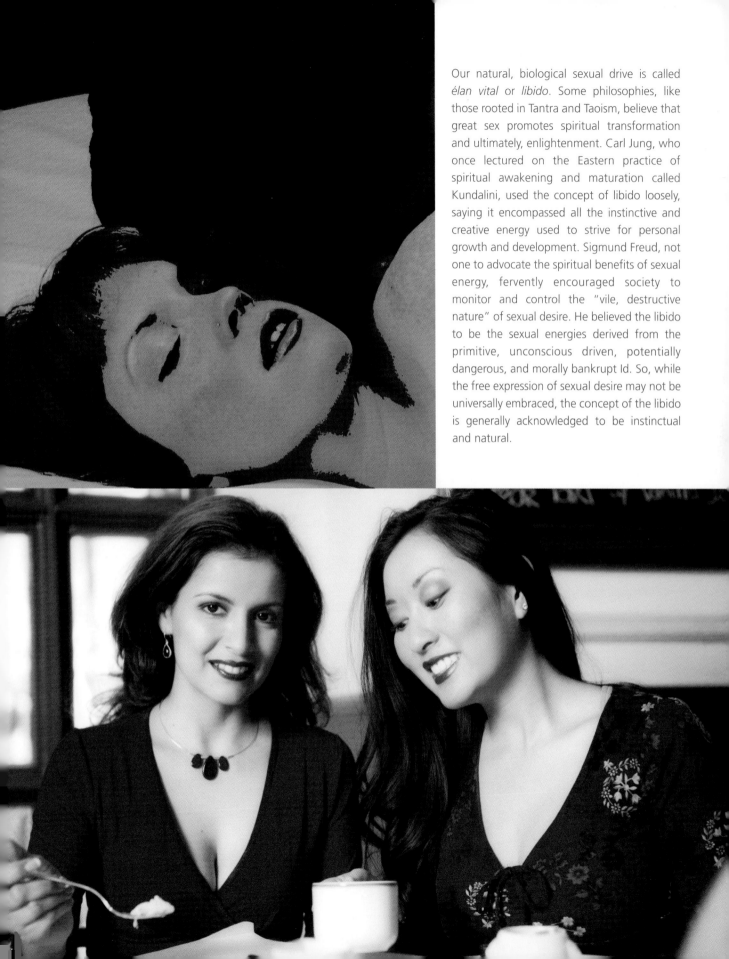

Our natural, biological sexual drive is called *élan vital* or *libido*. Some philosophies, like those rooted in Tantra and Taoism, believe that great sex promotes spiritual transformation and ultimately, enlightenment. Carl Jung, who once lectured on the Eastern practice of spiritual awakening and maturation called Kundalini, used the concept of libido loosely, saying it encompassed all the instinctive and creative energy used to strive for personal growth and development. Sigmund Freud, not one to advocate the spiritual benefits of sexual energy, fervently encouraged society to monitor and control the "vile, destructive nature" of sexual desire. He believed the libido to be the sexual energies derived from the primitive, unconscious driven, potentially dangerous, and morally bankrupt Id. So, while the free expression of sexual desire may not be universally embraced, the concept of the libido is generally acknowledged to be instinctual and natural.

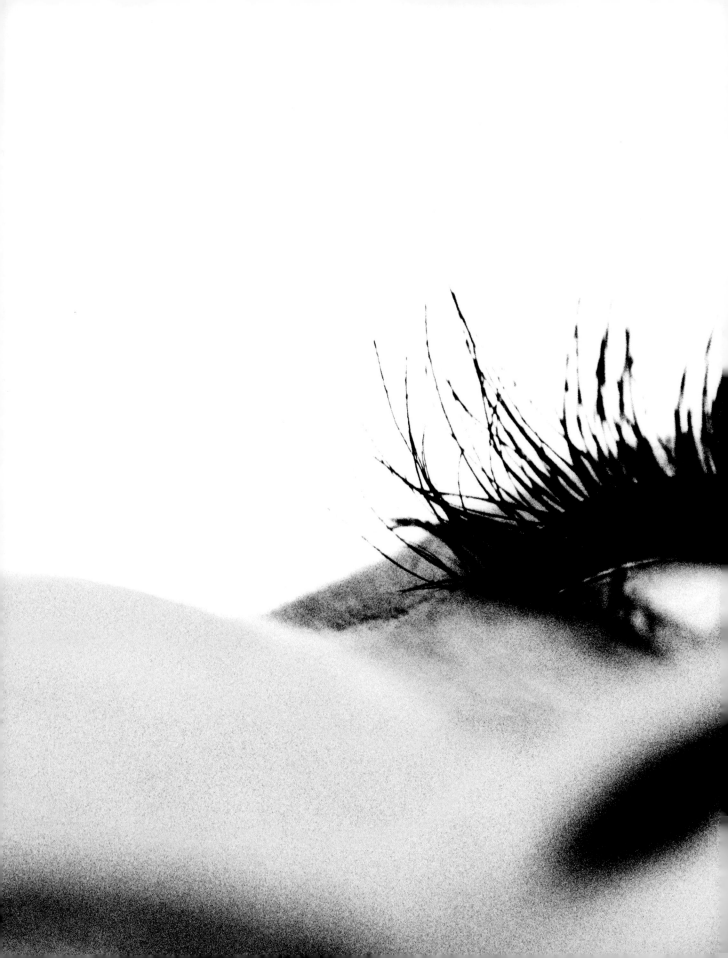

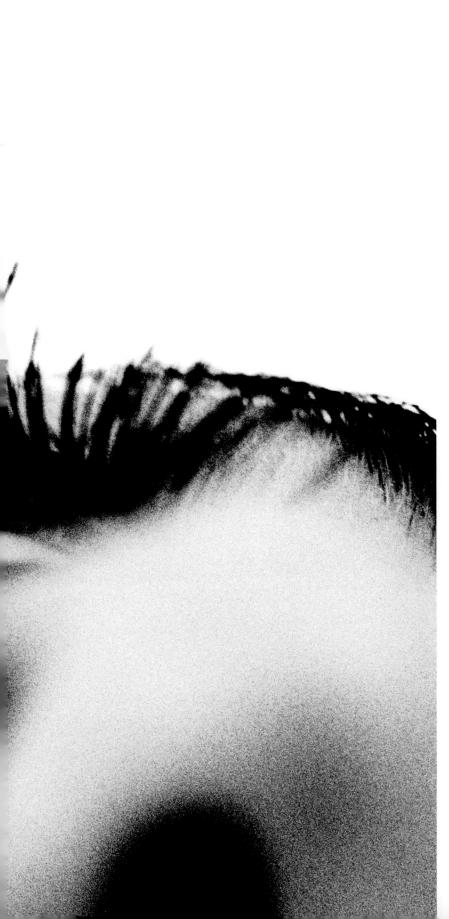

Romance begins with longing. There's a bounty of wonderful women out there, so much pleasure to be had and love to be shared. Why are we drawn to a particular woman at a particular point in time? Desire is born of attraction. Attraction usually begins with her physical attributes: how she looks, smells, sounds, and moves. We respond to symmetry and good posture, and although the mass media seems obsessed with the idea that attractiveness is synonymous with or heavily reliant upon youthfulness, it's not about youth, it is about health. Taste is highly relative, but in general, we are drawn to radiance, apparent in specific visual traits such as soft, shiny hair and glowing skin. Intelligence, ambition, a positive attitude and outlook on life, a sense of humor, and other indications of inner health and strength also ignite our desire to be with a particular woman.

Fantasy feeds the fire of desire and opposites occasionally attract, but a woman tends to be drawn to a woman whose style, taste, and perception of the world blend comfortably with her own. This validation of basic values, beliefs, and lifestyle choices, and the ensuing boost of confidence are crucial to fueling desire.

The emotional, physical, and spiritual booty from satisfied sexual desires are boundless, as long as one remembers that desire is dynamic. To experience and sustain sexual satisfaction we must keep a clear head while embracing the power of our natural libido, and acknowledge that through the years we will lead a dynamic sex life. This holds true whether you prefer multiple partners or are a one-woman woman. We are products of our experience, therefore what we find attractive changes as we ourselves develop and our tastes and priorities transform. Know and embrace the fact that what you want, and how and when you want it, will change. To deny this is to deny true gratification for both yourself and your lover or lovers.

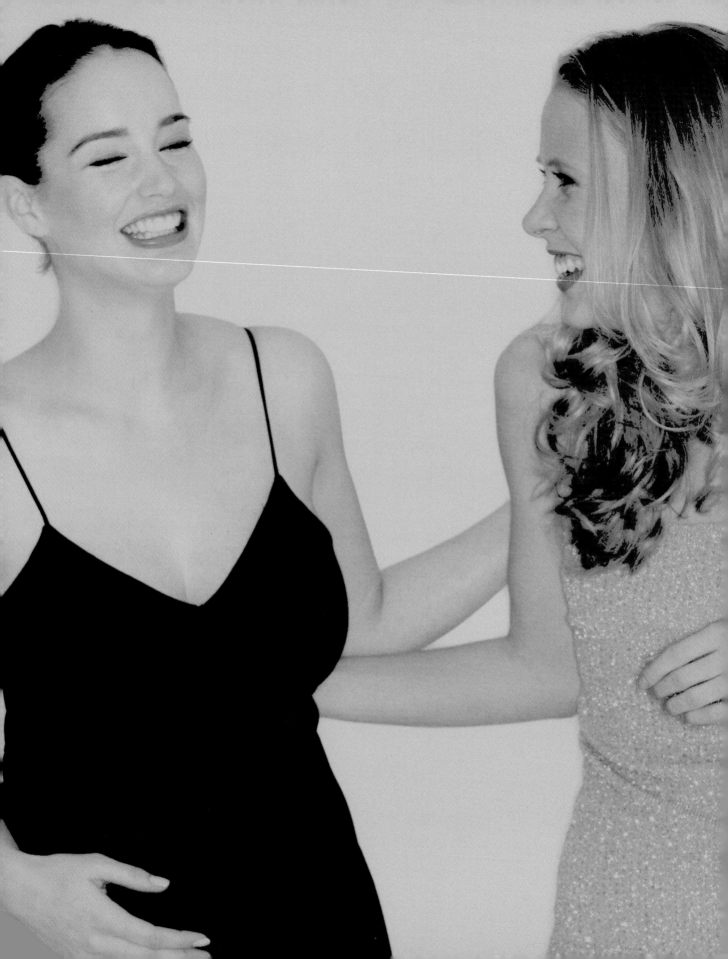

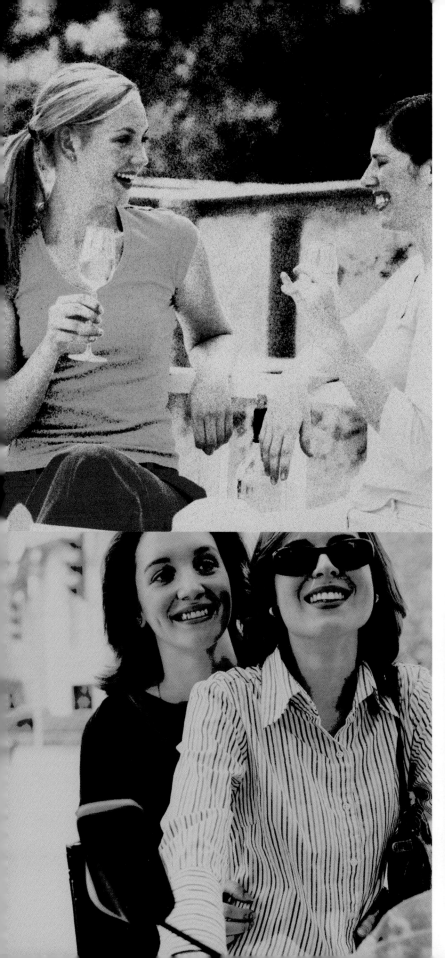

Sexual desire must be ignited to evolve into arousal. What turns her on? What arouses you? You may imagine that you are into spanking, so she slaps your bare bottom with her hairbrush and tells you how naughty you are, but it doesn't turn you on–it only makes you laugh. On the other hand, you had no idea how turned-on you would be when she came home from shopping, led you into the bedroom, and tied you to the headboard with her new silk scarf. Be adventurous, playful, and willing to evolve.

Physical characteristics of sexual arousal include increased heart rate, eye movements, and vasocongestion, otherwise known as the blushing and flushing of the skin. When we're really stirred up, our body anticipates amplified sexual activity and our breasts swell and nipples become erect, inviting more stimulation. The vagina expands and becomes moist and the vulva, in particular the clitoris, and inner labia swell. Sexual arousal may be characterized behaviorally by giddiness, incessant talking about your newfound love interest, the loss of the ability to listen to anyone about anything other than your newfound love interest, daydreaming, and the inability to focus, singing in the streets, and frequent fantasizing.

When we first met she preferred to be kissed aggressively, French kissed, combined with mutual groping, especially of each others' breasts. After a bit of this she'd lie on her back and spread her legs for oral sex. As I licked her she would plead for my fingers to simultaneously penetrate her swelling pussy, and then she'd climax. Over time the routine, as satisfying as it always was became, well, routine. Now, years later, we've discovered we're both really into her lying on her stomach with me straddling and rubbing on her backside, teasingly whispering my 'dirty' intentions into her ear as I tie her hands above her head with a silk scarf. She becomes so wet that I actually wipe away some of her moisture onto my midriff before inserting the dildo. As I penetrate her I reach underneath and rub her clit until she climaxes, the first of many times.

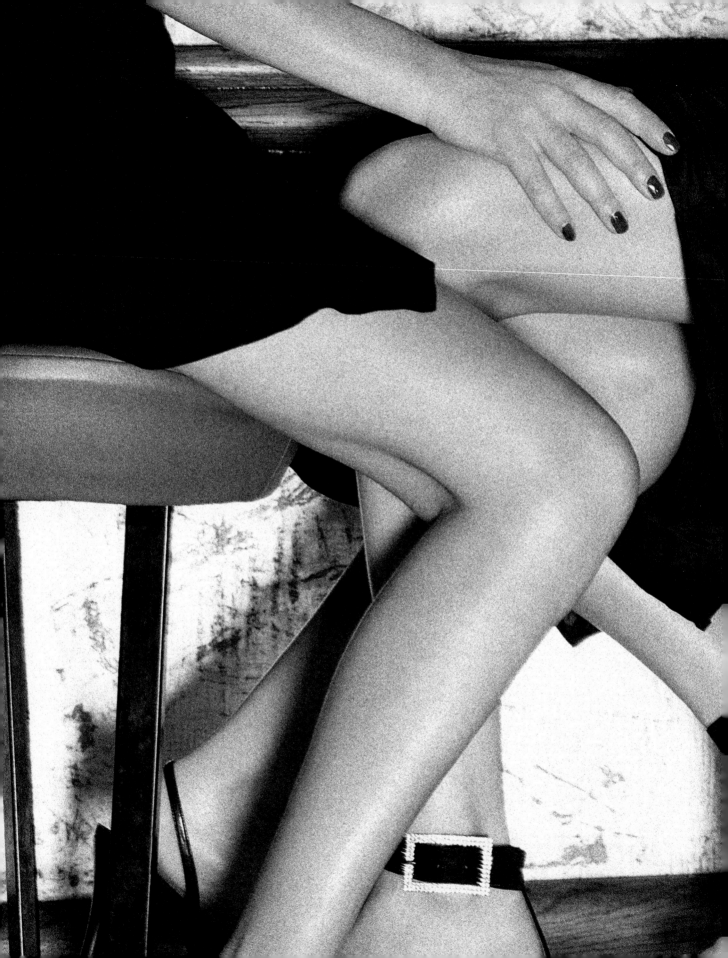

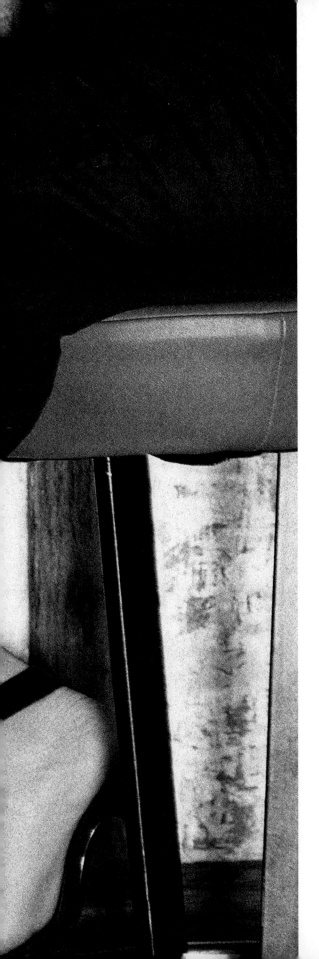

Flirting is a way to express attraction and attractiveness, desire and desirability. "To flirt" is derived from the old French "conter fleurette;" an attempt to seduce by the dropping of flower petals. If you don't have flower petals readily available, intrigue her with direct eye contact, entice her with a smile, make her laugh with your wit, and excite her with a wink.

flirt

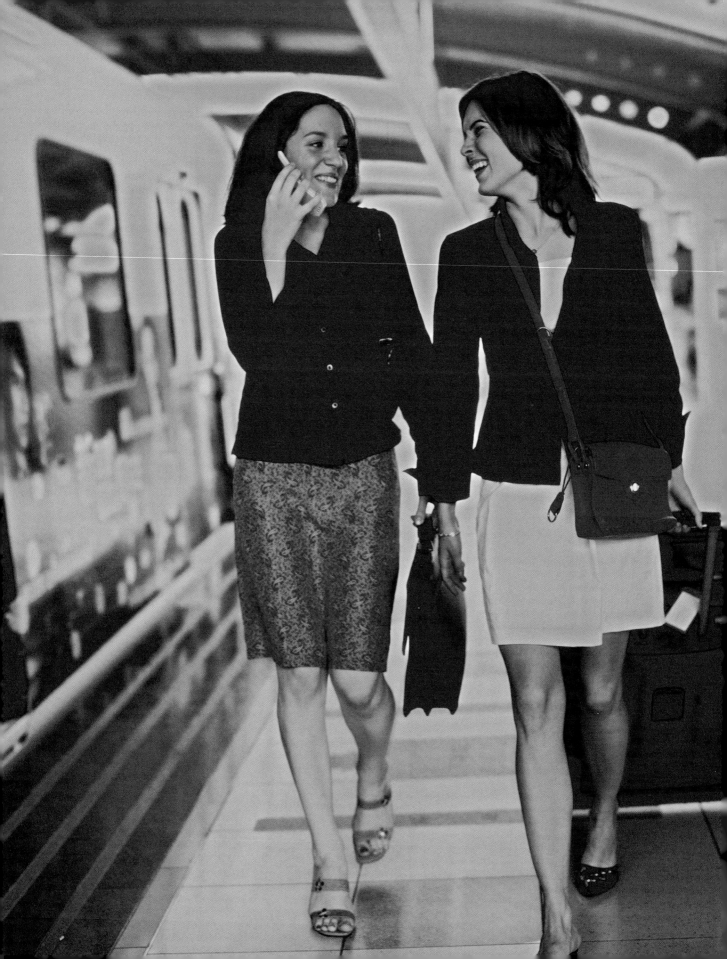

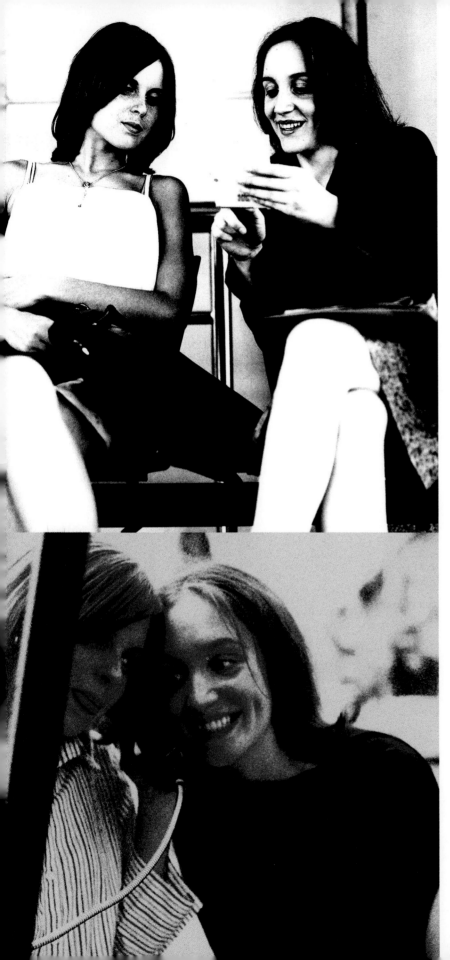

Flirting is a casual and socially acceptable form of interaction that allows us to determine our level and type of interest in another woman. Flirting doesn't always say, "I want you," but it does communicate a desire to connect, and often it's the desire to connect sexually. We don't sleep with everyone we flirt with. We do flirt with those we like or are drawn to, whether or not our conscious intention is seduction.

Flirting allows us to test the waters of desire. You see someone across the room and are immediately attracted to her, so you watch her, discreetly at first, and interpret further her character based on visual clues. After watching her for a bit, you may decide your first impression was off-base and that you are no longer interested, or the desire to know her may grow, so you bolster the courage and approach her. Again, further interaction may or may not solidify our initial impressions, but it isn't until we somehow make contact that we determine what sort of relationship we are interested in pursuing.

Flirting is a skill that can be developed and honed. Notice what draws you to flirt with someone. Is it her sense of humor? Does the shape of her neck make you hot for her? Her PhD? The small of her back? When you touch her arm flirtatiously does your spark of desire grow into arousal?

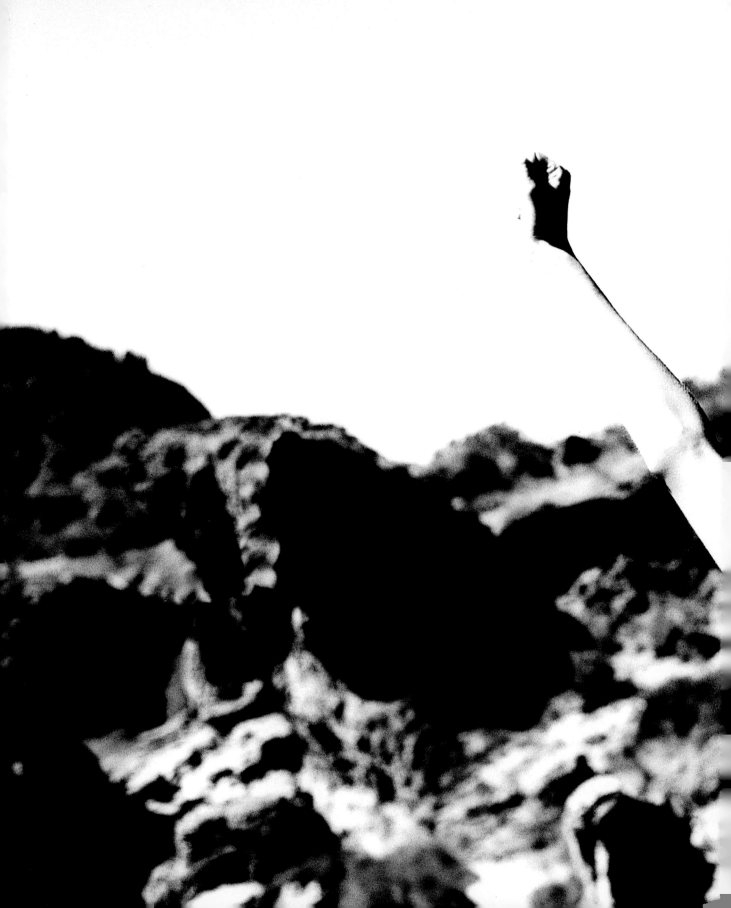

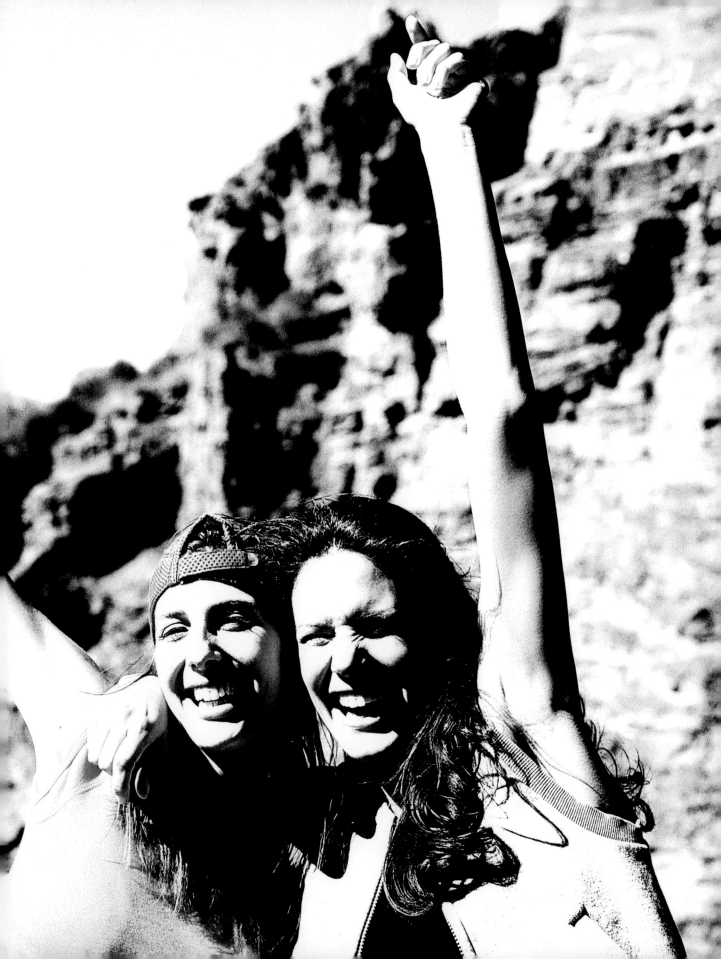

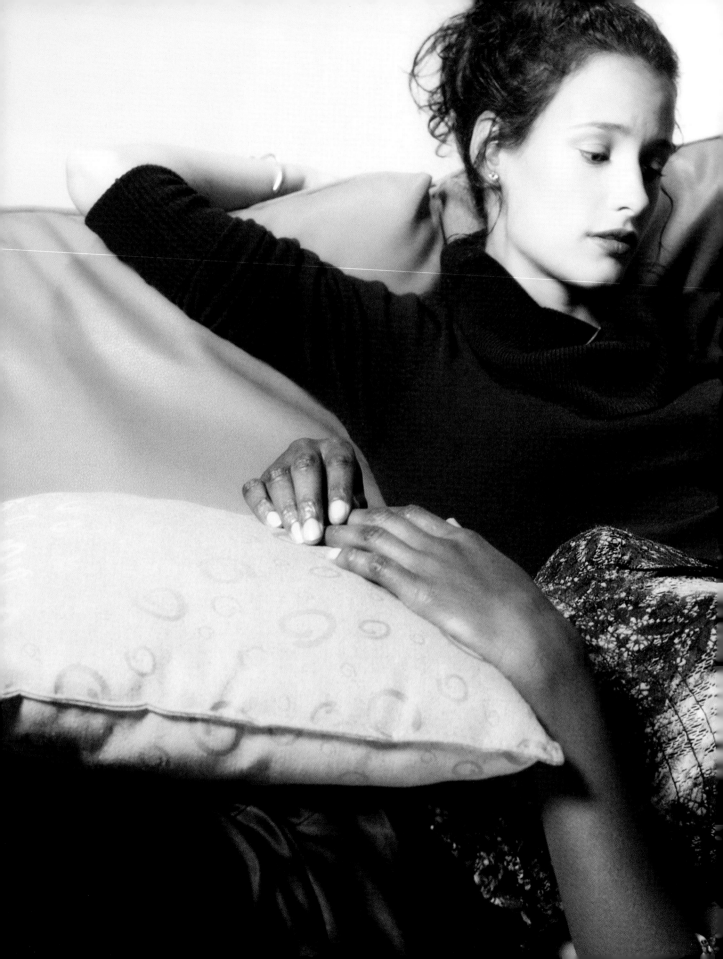

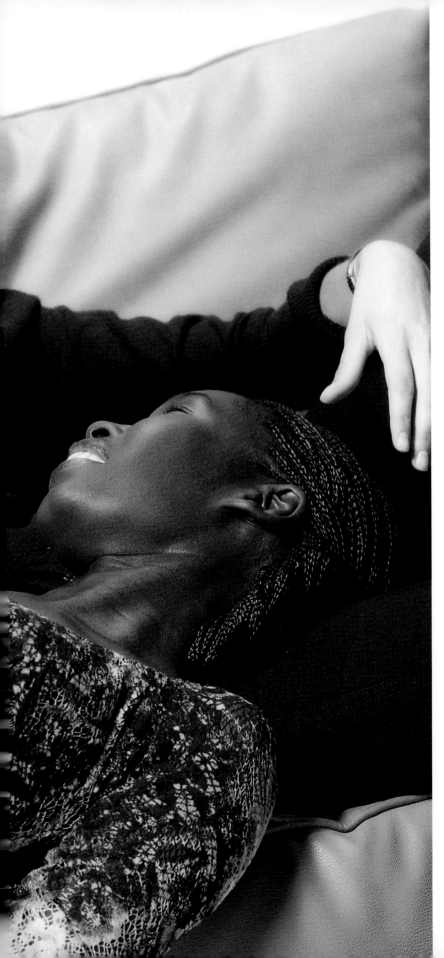

Practice flirting. Play off of what draws you to her to gain her attention. Tell her how great her leather jacket is, then tell her how great she looks while wearing it and that few women could do it the same justice. Charm and sincerity will persuade her that you are worthy of her consideration.

Incite her imagination. Again, language is one of the finest flirting tools. Keep on top of current events and be armed with a few clever quotes or lines of snappy dialogue. Double entendres have managed to entertain us through the ages. A slight indelicacy may amuse her. And a timely and well–delivered sampling of your particular sensibility will speak volumes. In the words of Mae West, "it's better to be looked over than overlooked."

A titillating turn-on is to tease. The most satisfying tease occurs when a woman actually gives the recipient of the tease what she desires, but very, very slowly. Teasing as a prelude to the main event requires the perfect combination of agony and pleasure. Much of the popularity of burlesque and the striptease is related to the thrill of being gradually seduced.

Don't stop flirting when you are in bed. Elicit unusual sensations by having your lover lie back and close her eyes, then with your finger "write" racy messages on her midriff. Make her guess what you're writing and proceed accordingly.

The ability to gain and maintain a woman's attention is essential to a pleasurable sex life. Flirting doesn't stop once you've hooked your prey. Everyday flirting in a relationship benefits both partners. Playfulness, mutual enjoyment, and laughter induce hormones to continually flush our spirits with good feelings.

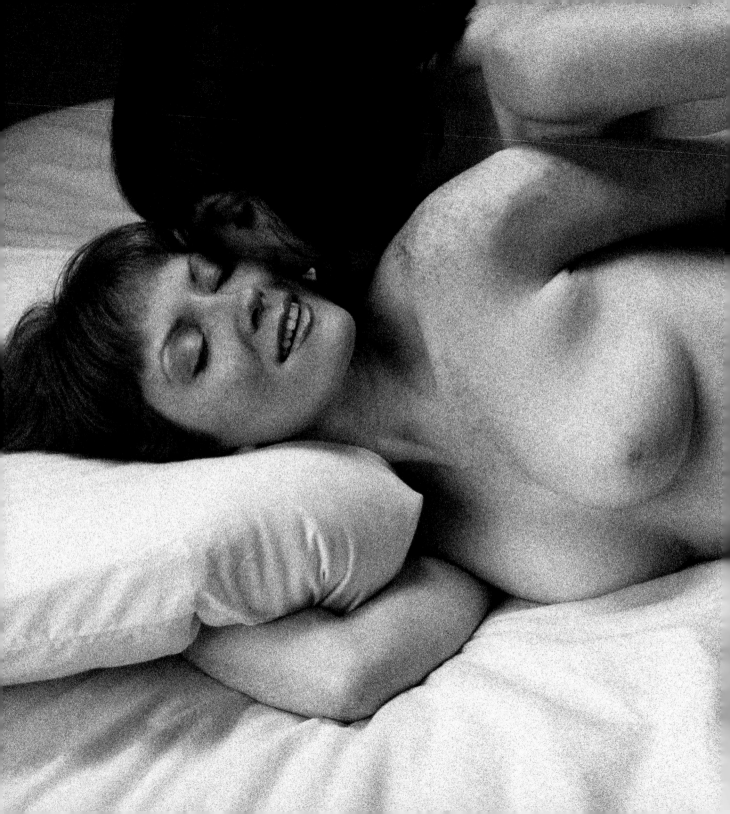

scent

The olfactory sense is a key player in the biology of attraction and seduction.

Pheromones, from the Greek "pherein" (to carry), and "hormone" (to excite) are inexplicably powerful attractants. Generated by the apocrine glands, pheromones instantly communicate whether we like or dislike someone. Although the specifics are widely disputed, pheromones are generally accepted to be the naturally occurring chemicals and virtually undetectable aromas we secrete.

Through the sense of smell, the tiniest bit of pheromones can communicate messages about danger and turf or territory, food and fertility, but most interesting, the reaction is basically copulatory— "I want you, whoever you are that's secreting that chemical and making me all love–crazy!"

Some researchers believe the pheromone's transmission is received by the vomeronasal organ (VNO), a chemoreceptive structure located at the base of the nasal septum. Others dispute the existence or function of the VNO in humans or even whether pheromones affect humans. But it is indisputable that the power of sexual attraction can be surprisingly strong and at times inexplicable.

Humans are capable of scent memory. Smell shares its part of the cerebral cortex with memory and emotion, two mental faculties that are not touted as the most sensible parts of our nature. Although the scent memories we retain may not always be rooted in rationality, their power is indisputable. The smell of the ocean, a spice, or a particular perfume can immediately provoke thoughts of a childhood at the sea, a broken heart, or your first love.

Light a candle scented with ylang–ylang and cypress when you next make love. This sweet scent will forever remind you and your lover of one another.

I am totally overwhelmed by her. I can't believe it because she's totally not my typical taste in women, but I don't think of anything or anyone else. Yesterday when she passed by me she touched my shoulder and smiled. Every nerve ending in my body quivered. I noticed my shoulder had this subtle scent of jasmine where her hand had been. I asked her what she was wearing and promptly bought the same perfume. She was flattered. Of course when I wear, it I think of her.

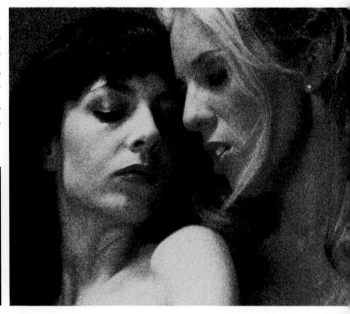

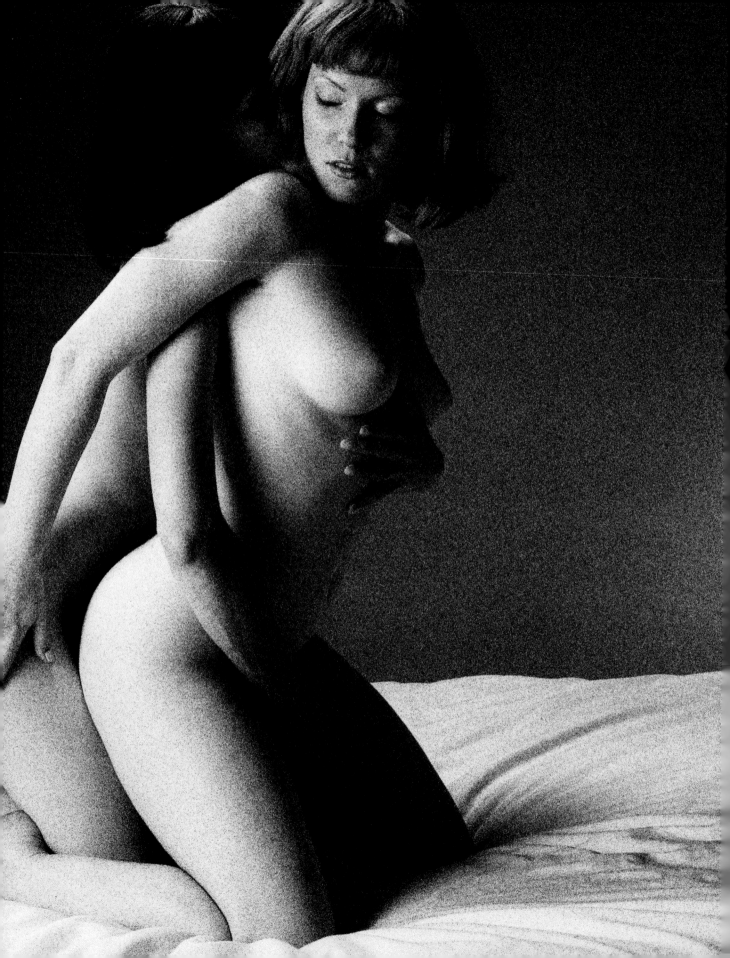

Touch nurtures us throughout our lives. Fulfilling our basic need for affection and human contact, touch helps us develop sexually, socially, and psychologically. Indeed, touching and being touched benefits our overall health. Placing a hand on a woman's shoulder, whether a surprise, soft, heavy, or lingering touch, can say "trust me," "hey, settle down!" or "I like you." A touch from the right woman can make you swoon, but toucher beware, as even the most fleeting touch can have a dramatic, and lasting influence.

touch

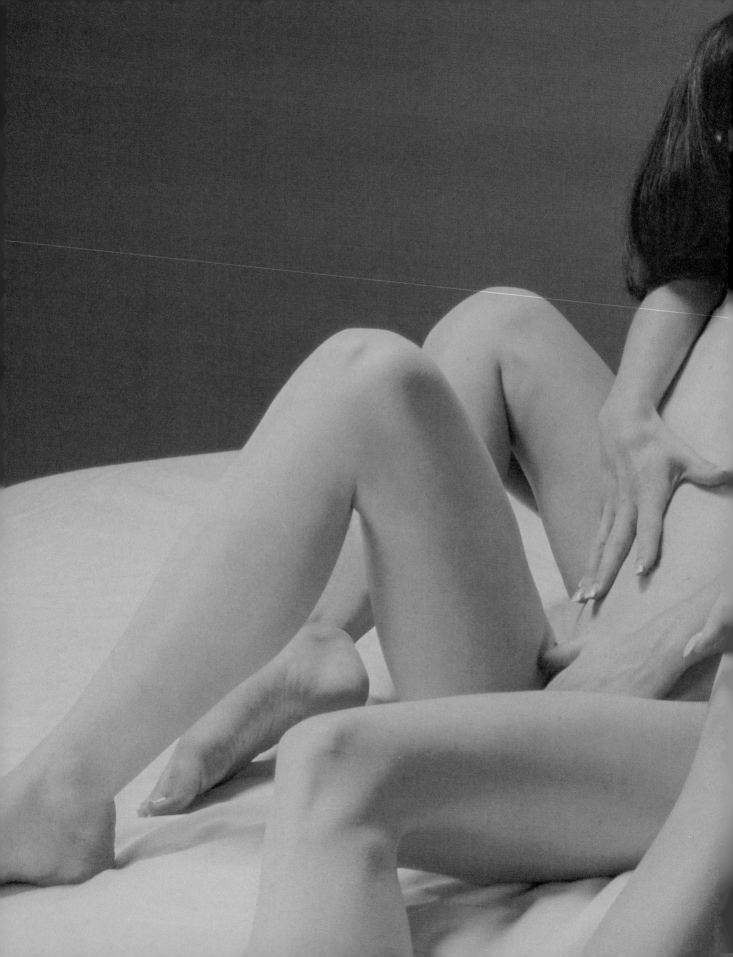

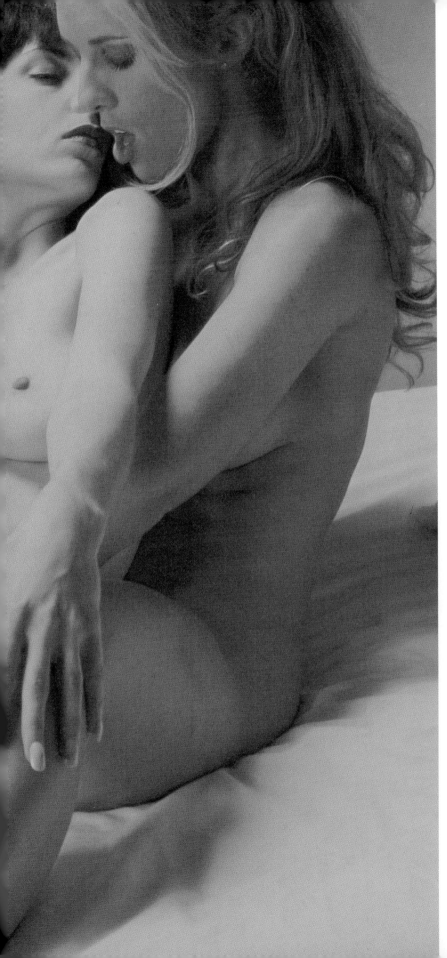

Most sexual exploration happens with touch. Discover your lover's sexual landscape; her shapes and soft, smooth, firm, and silky textures from top to bottom. Every woman's body is more or less sensitive in different areas, at different times. Highly sensitive areas include the lips, the tip of the tongue, the face, neck, earlobes, feet, fingertips, under the arms, and the tender backs of the knees.

Touching is an intimate act that involves a great deal of trust. In fact, we ourselves may not know what we want or how vulnerable certain bodily contact may make us feel until the game is underway. A woman may want to be caressed softly one night and fucked hard the next. Although mutual, open communication is always encouraged, don't expect a woman to verbalize or otherwise articulate her preferences and moods. Be receptive to interpreting her body language to make sure your touch is eliciting the desired response.

Massage relaxes us and encourages openness, and can be practiced before, during, and after sex. Heating up her skin utilizing massage-type body exploration will make her more receptive to your touch. Pressing your palm onto a woman conveys a deeper, more commanding desire that establishes or reinforces power relations and negotiates levels of intimacy. Respect one another's boundaries and unique capacities and desires to partake in varying levels of intimacy.

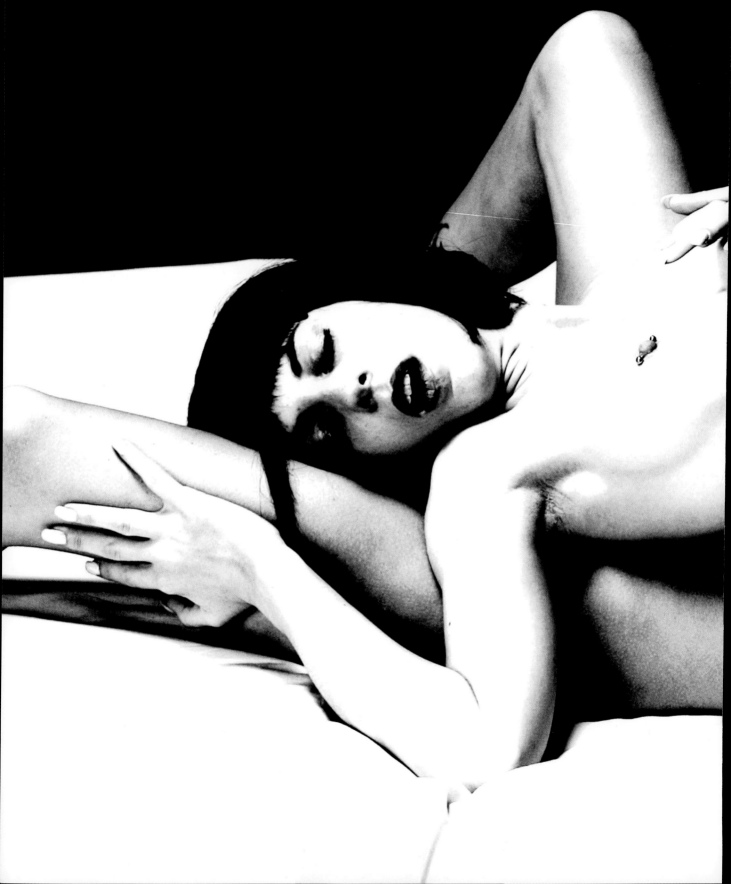

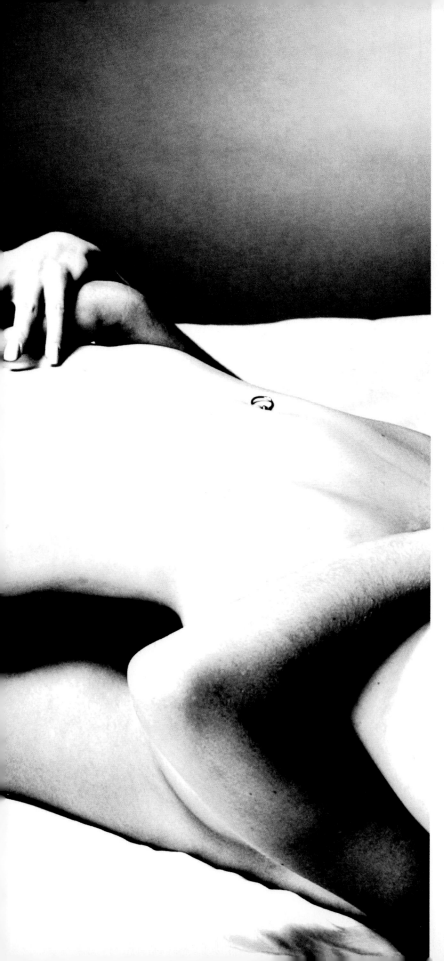

As lovers become comfortable with the touch of their partner, sensory experiments can heighten the sexual experience. Sensory deprivation challenges the typical responses of both your body and mind. Mix it up by having your lover wear a blindfold. Hesitate as she wonders when or where the next sensation will strike, then surprise her with a warm or cold touch. The sensations of heat and cold can be startling and invigorating. Trace her nipple with an ice cube, continuing along her quivering body until the cube melts.

Maintain a sense of humor in your sex life and with your sexual identity. Tickling produces laughter, which releases euphoric brain chemicals like endorphins, dopamine, and adrenaline. Excessive tickling is more torture than fun, so remember, tickle lightly, perhaps with a feather, for the most pleasurable experience.

For some sexual escapades, slow, focused exploration helps new or experimenting sexual partners to overcome inhibitions. Slow also builds anticipation. Take your time. Prolong the play until she is so aroused that it becomes unbearable and she demands that you set her free and bring her to climax to release her built-up sexual energy.

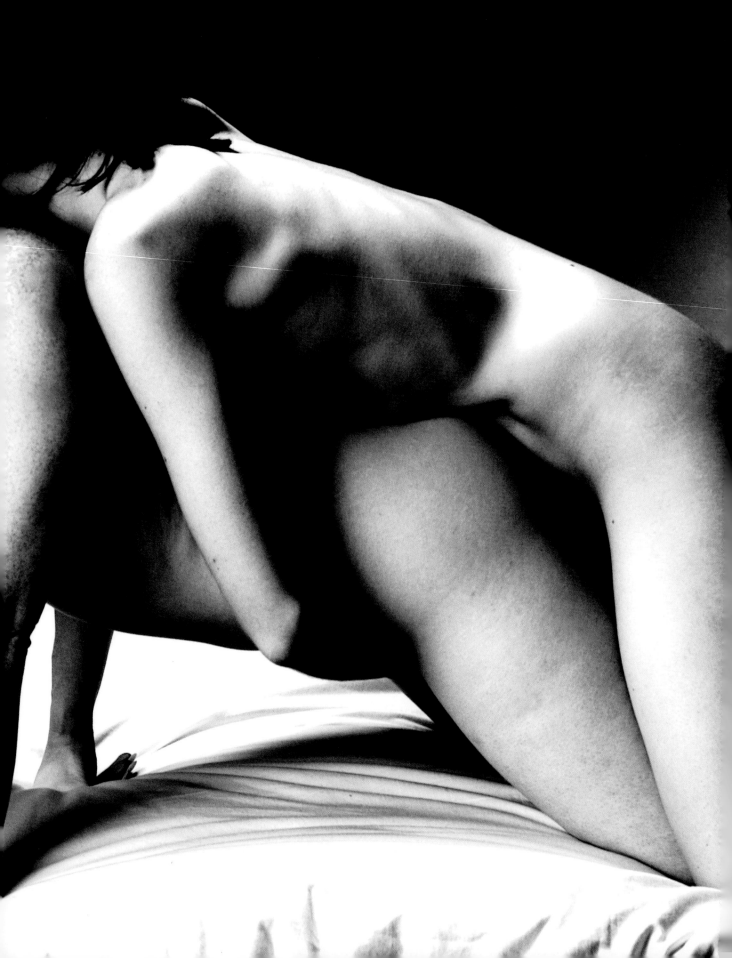

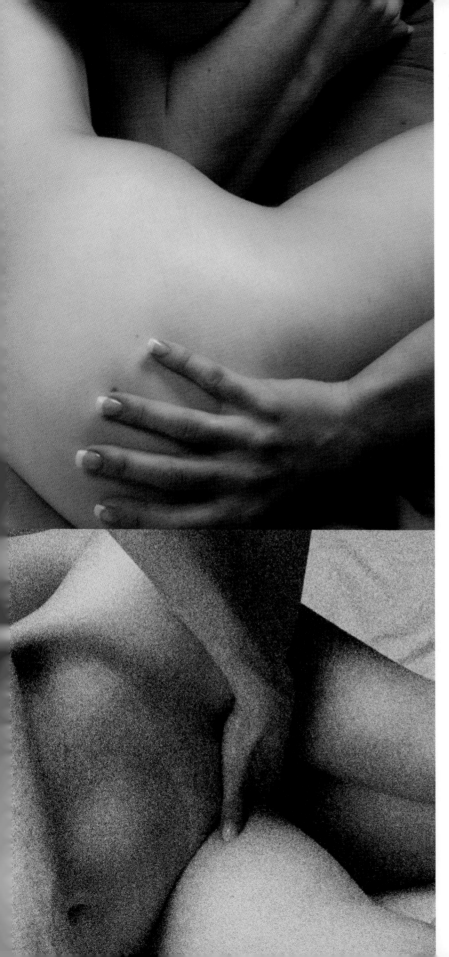

Equally as exciting can be fast, groping, more aggressive foreplay. If you cannot wait to touch her all over, don't. It may suit the mood and will certainly establish the tone and rhythm for the rest of the encounter.

Girl-wrapping is a playful bit of wrestling, a subtle power game, which ignites energy and heightens the desire for more. When you mount another woman, you'll discover that many parts of your body can touch various areas of hers. Wrap your legs around your lover and grind your pussy against her skin. This is exciting for both women and conveys both trust and lust as you spread your legs to expose your vulva before pressing it against her.

As women's bodies meld together in a soft crush, surely the labia is swelling and she's wet. Passion begins to consume, nipples are touched, tugged even and then pressed together, breast to breast. Stay close and navigate the path to her pussy. Touch her there. The vulva can be cupped, circled with a finger, tickled, and stroked. Think outside the box; once trust is established, the possibilities of how and where women touch one another are endless.

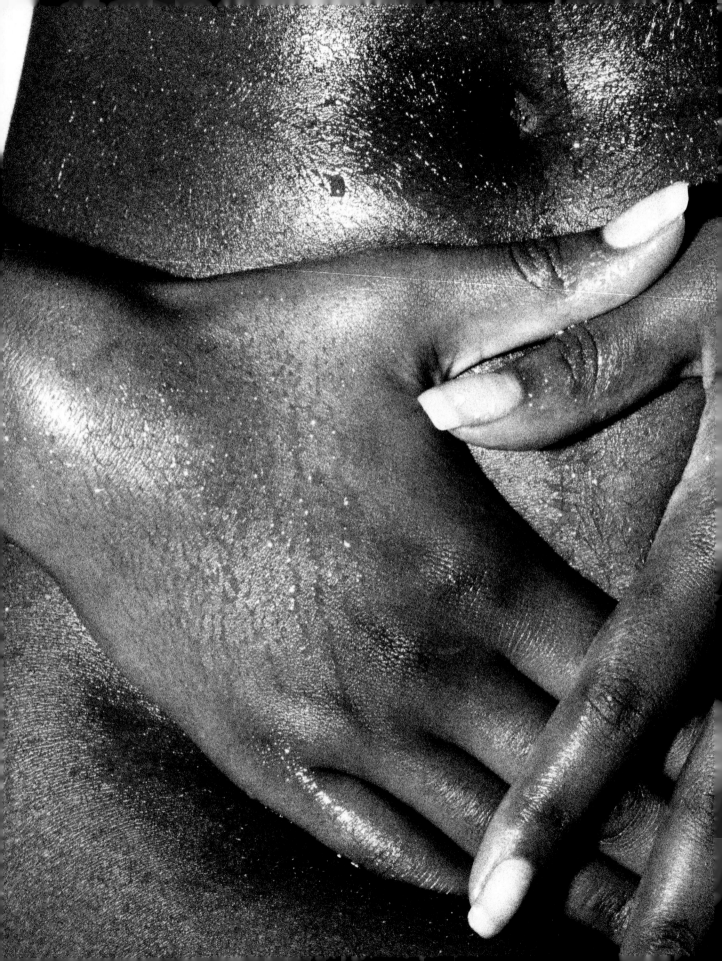

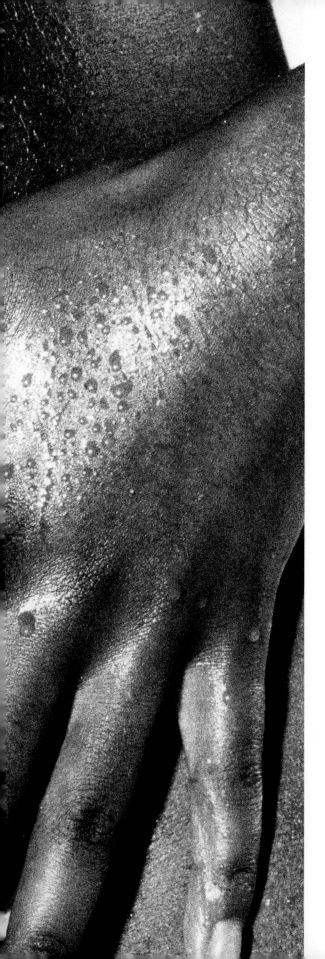

There is something comforting in being saturated. Perhaps it's the formative time spent in the womb that inspires us to seek moisture in various ways throughout our lives and water is, of course, essential to live. We take in and discharge all sorts of moistness—water, saliva, tears, sweat, and of course, the sexy self-lubricant the vagina emits as its walls become wet in anticipation of sexual activity. Wet is sexy.

wet

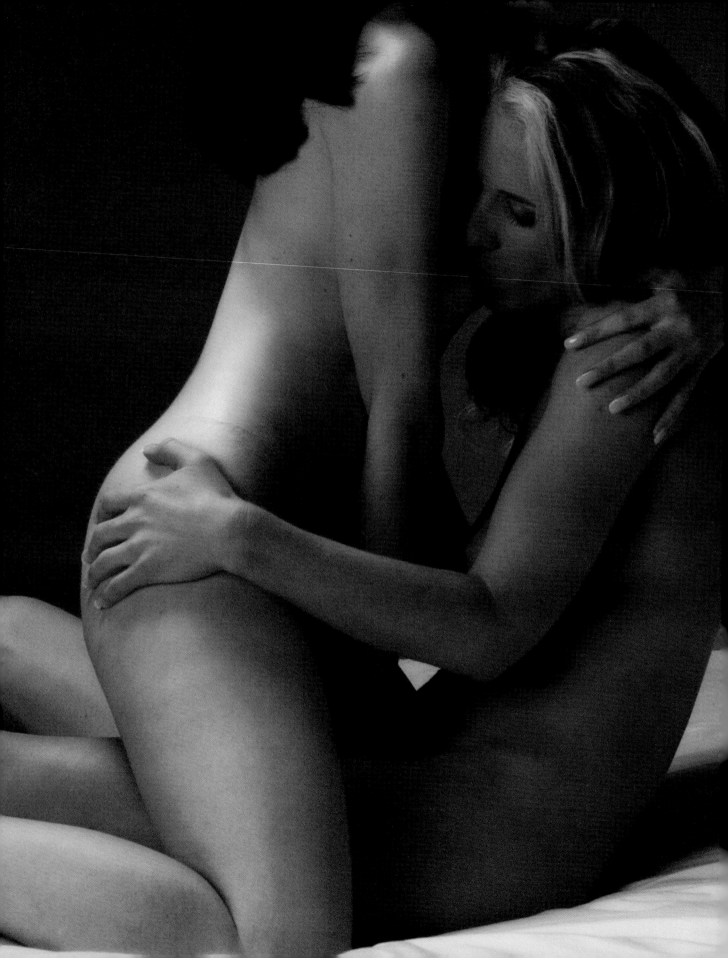

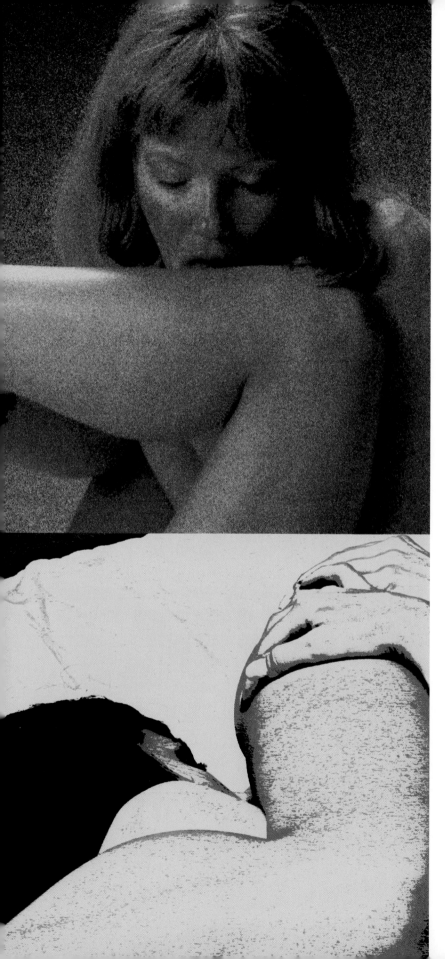

A kiss is often the first taste of another's moistness. Lips meet, tongues touch, and there's either a spark or a fizzle. Assuming a spark, your warm, wet mouth can continue beyond hers to trace the nape of her neck, circle her breast, and lick her nipple.

Dual sensations of wetness are particularly exhilarating. Give her a wet kiss while inserting your fingers inside her vagina. Wet your fingers in your mouth first if she's not yet moist enough for you to go deep inside. Take warm water into your mouth. After a moment, swallow most of it and then place your mouth onto her pussy.

For comfortable and pleasant vaginal penetration, it is essential that this tender region is wet. Incidentally, a woman's natural secretions are also the best, safest natural cleansers for the vagina. The amount of lubrication that is released naturally, which is affected by mood, hormones, and medicines to name a few, need not impact sexual pleasure. Many water-based and other lubricants are readily available through your local pharmacy or online and at stores like Babeland or Good Vibrations. Ask questions, do your research, and take into account whether or not the lube you want should be ingestible, hypoallergenic, or simply the right choice for each toy and intended sexual act.

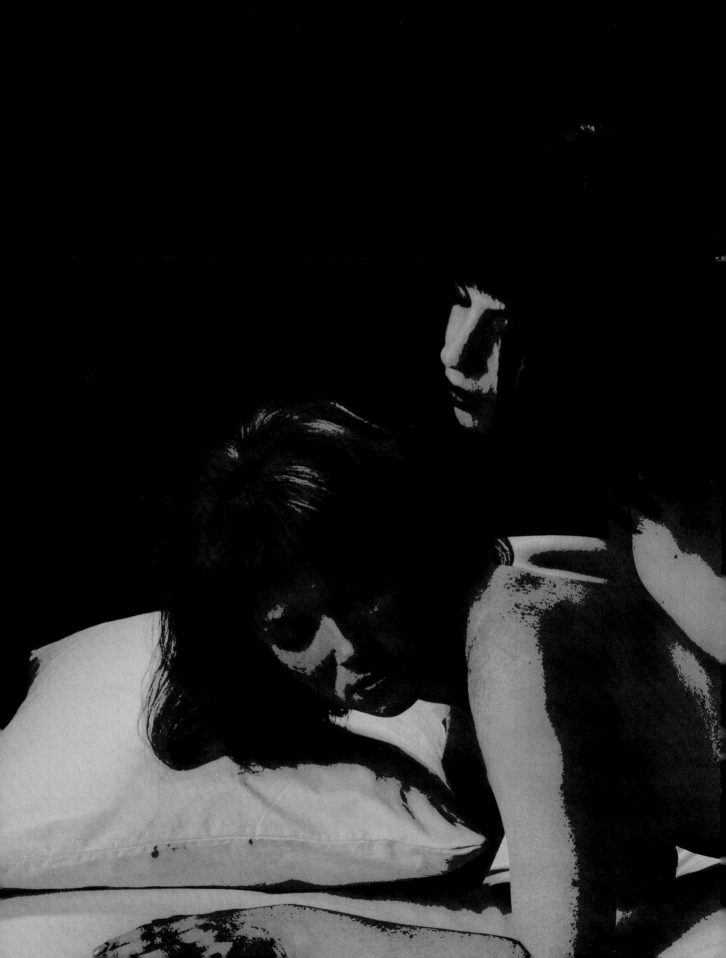

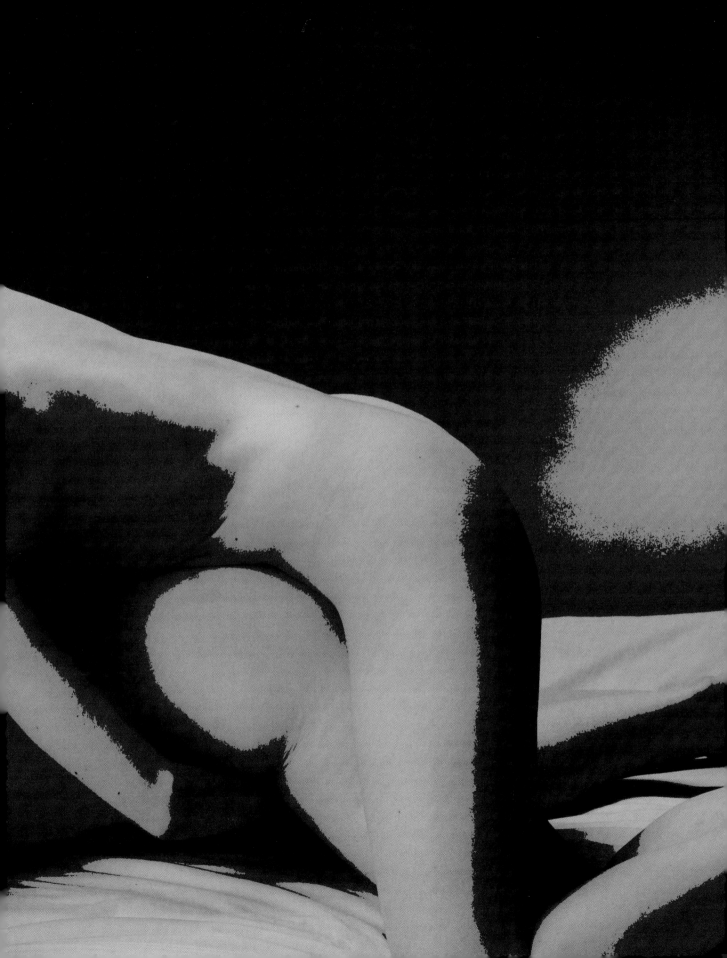

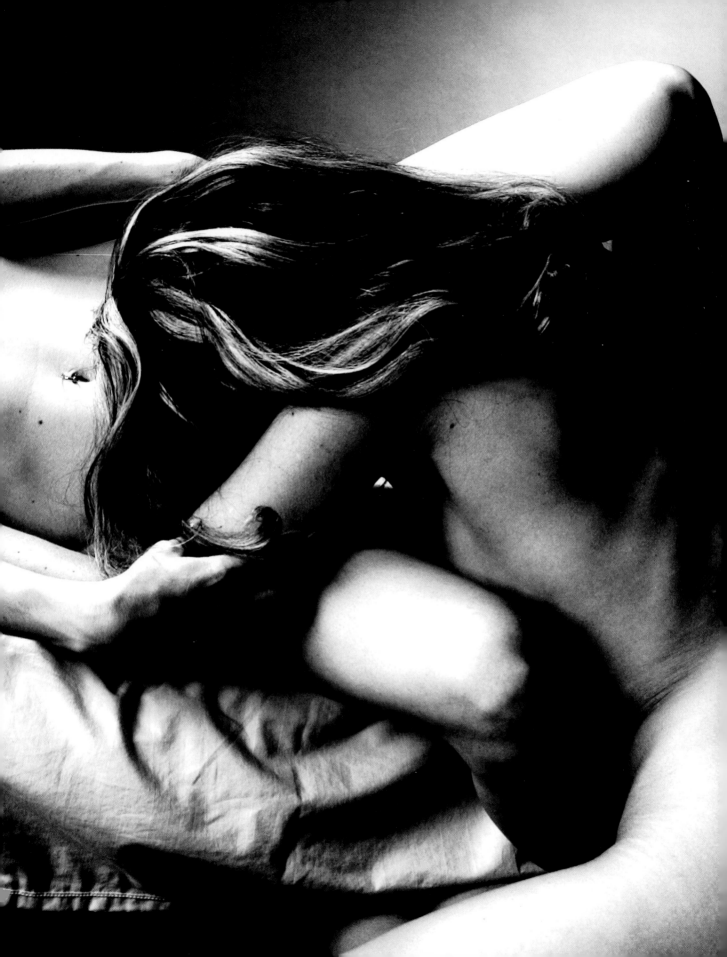

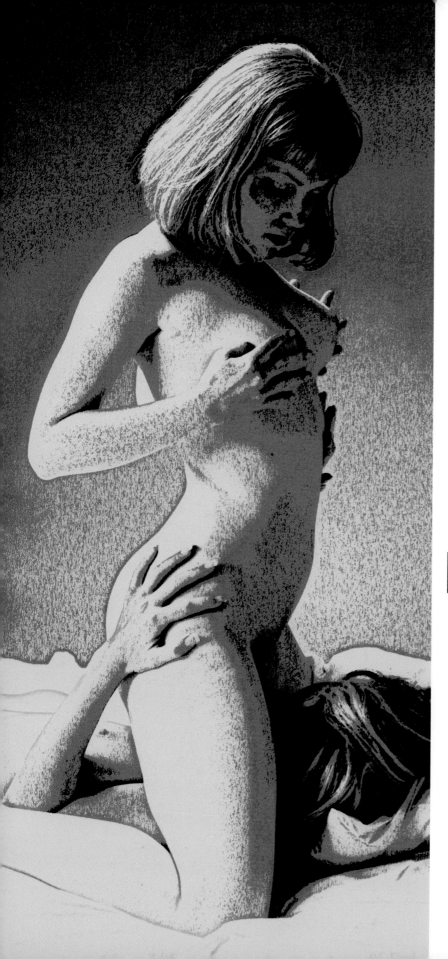

A superb prelude to prepare both women's bodies for a moist sex session is to incorporate massage into foreplay. Slick bodies make for a sexy lovemaking experience. Choose good quality massage oil and caress her shoulders, lower back, and buns. Once she is shimmering, climb on top, press your body onto hers, and slip and slide away.

One way to get wet and stay wet is to make love in a pool, shower, or while soaking together in a bath. Pulsating jets or the showerhead are practical accessories likened to waterproof vibrators. The wet, private arena of a personal spa is also an ideal environment to get to know and explore oneself, testing physical reactions to the touching and penetrating of different areas of your body.

Just as more lubrication is sometimes required, a woman can also be too wet for her ultimate enjoyment. Comfortable and truly satisfying sex involves texture and demands some friction. When one of you becomes exceedingly wet, sweep with your hand the dripping, swelling vagina and wipe that warm, silky, milky juice on the nearest glistening thigh.

> *Wow. You are so wet. Give me your hand. Here. Feel how wet you're making me.*

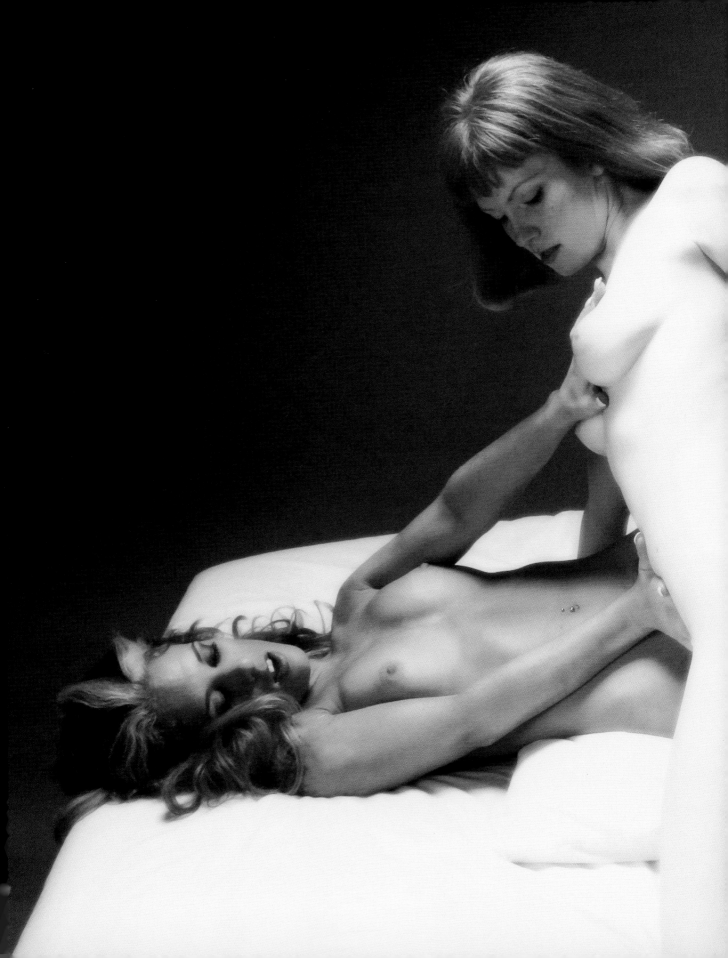

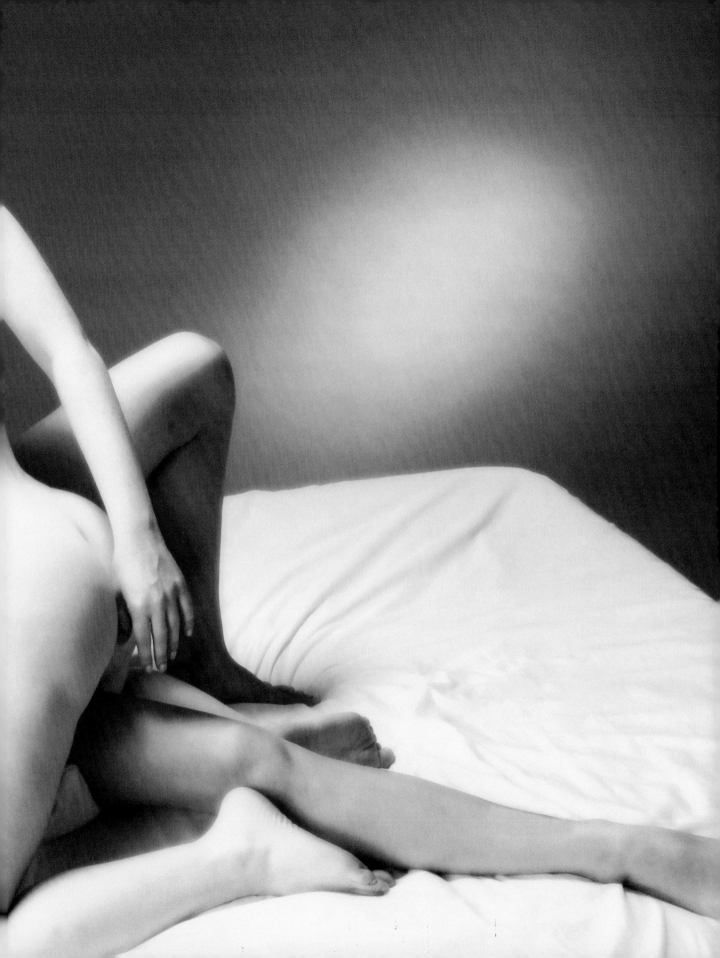

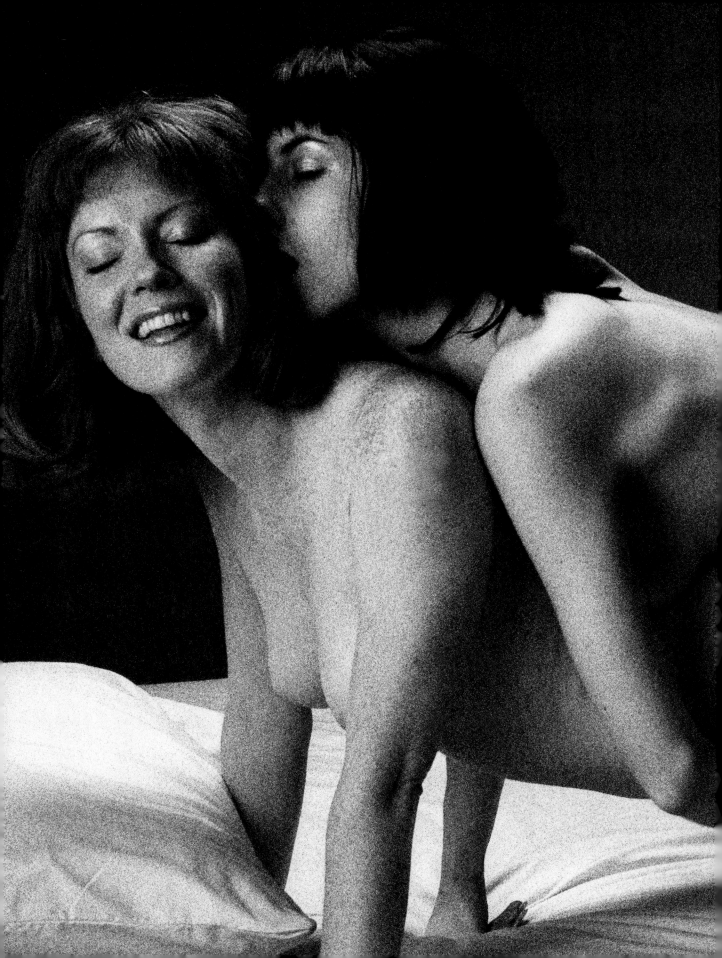

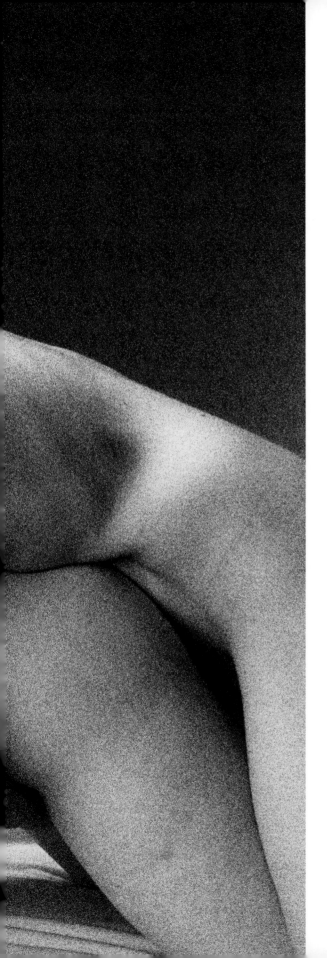

Small, gentle, intermittent nibbles greatly enhance lovemaking. The stimulation to our nerve endings incites tingling and increases our receptivity to upcoming sensations. The primal action of nibbling is not only a great way to express your desire to know her, but also a delicious way to physically explore your lover's every familiar curve and forbidden nook.

nibble

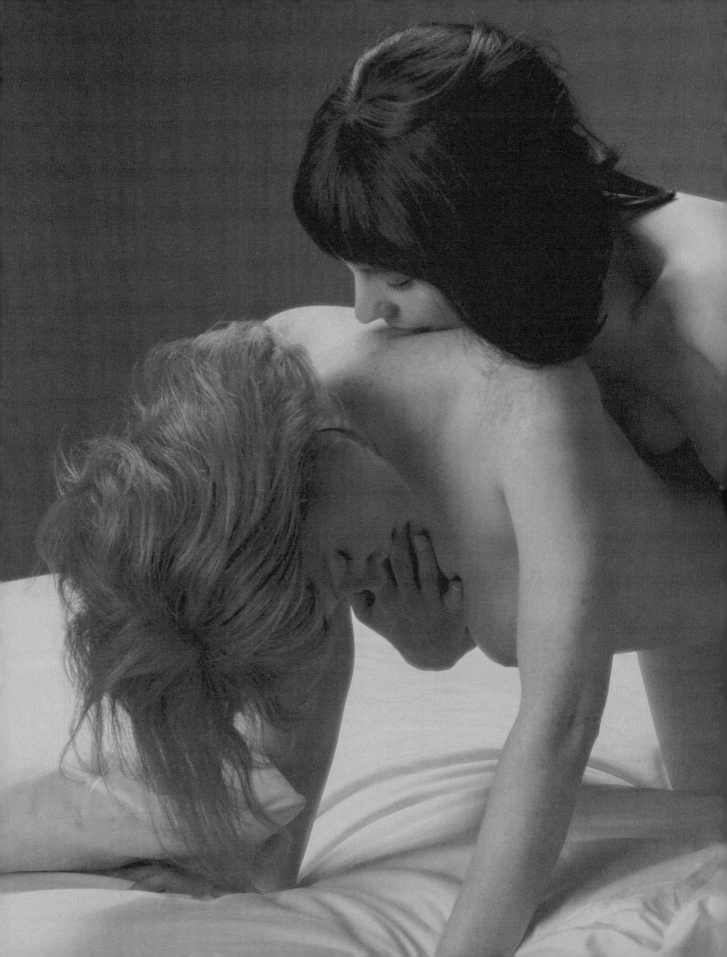

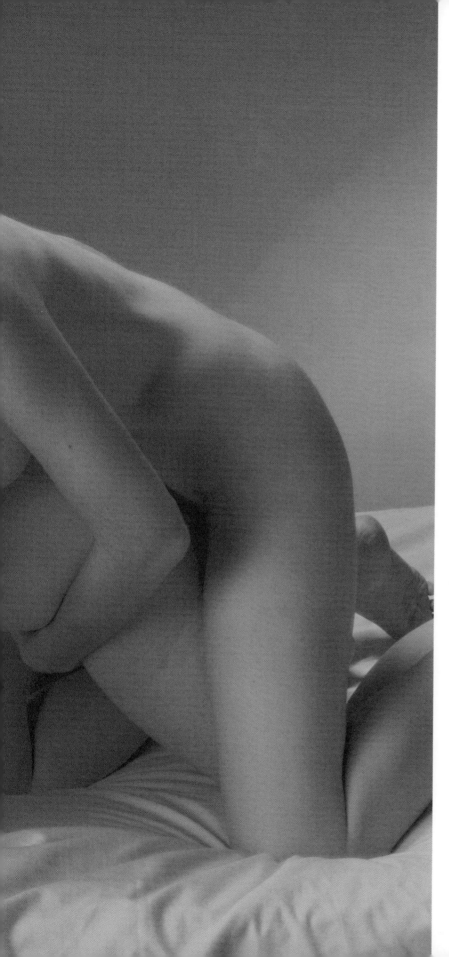

The female body is a nibble paradise. The mystifying seduction of the vampire has captivated us for years, largely because the neck is such a sexy stretch of skin. Embrace her from behind and lightly bite her shoulder, upper back, or nosh on her neck. This will send chills throughout her body, and her nipples will harden and become erect. Nibbling heightens the anticipation for both lovers as the excitement it provokes increases feelings of anxiousness and sexual hunger. It often leads to a more aggressive and exhilarating lovemaking session.

Like the clitoris and vaginal and anal regions, a stimulated nipple fills with blood, swells and becomes erect, rendering it and the area around the nipple particularly receptive to any extra attention. Just as she is climaxing, lightly but firmly clamp down on her nipple. This move requires exquisite timing, but the resulting orgasm will be especially sweet.

Part of the impact of nibbling is attributable to the passion and dash of danger involved. To trust someone to be as intimate as to nibble, touch, kiss, and lick every inch of your body takes courage. Trust indicates to a partner that you believe you can rely on her, that she has integrity, and that you are confident in her abilities as a lover.

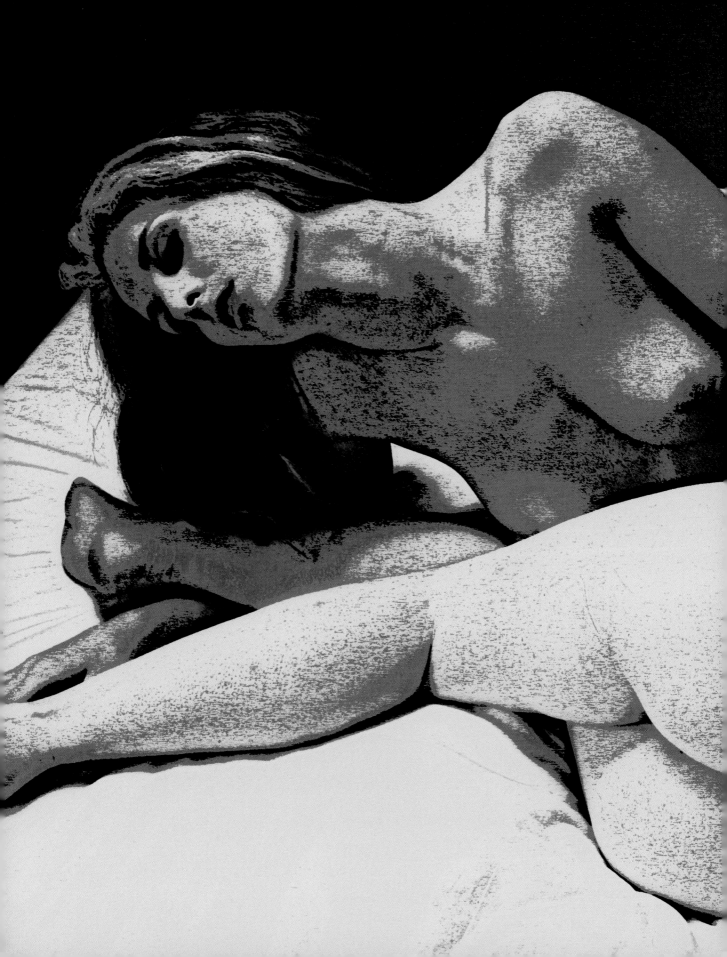

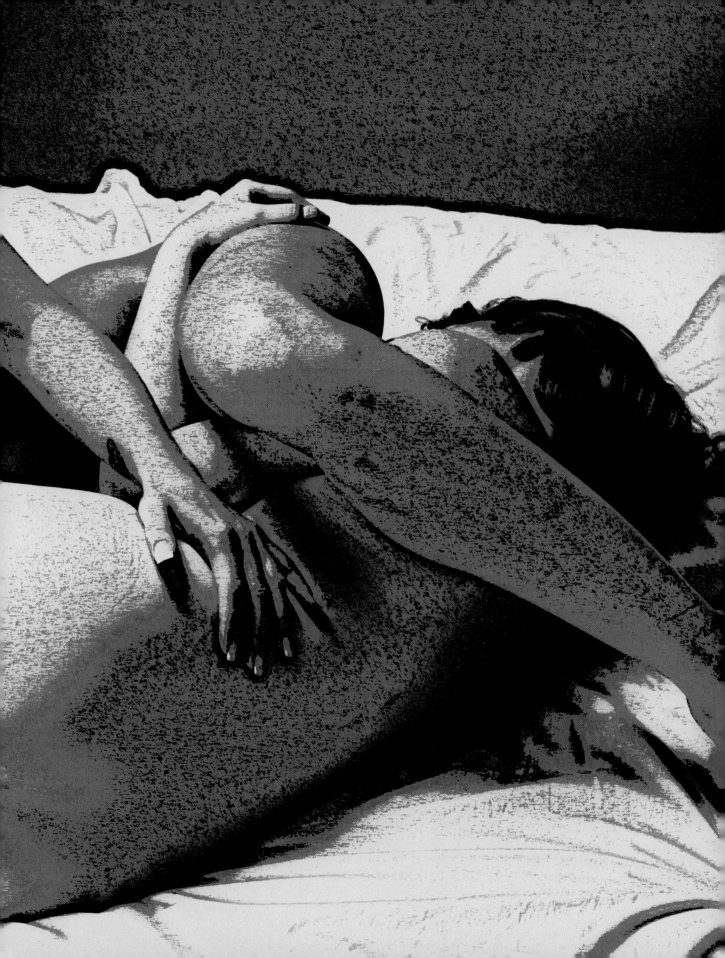

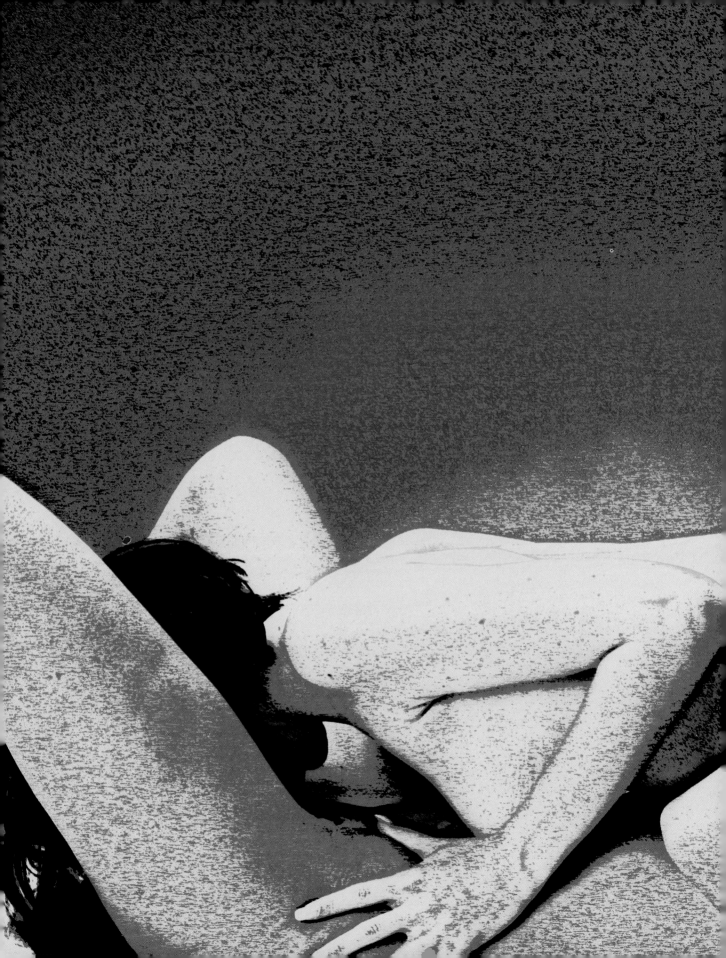

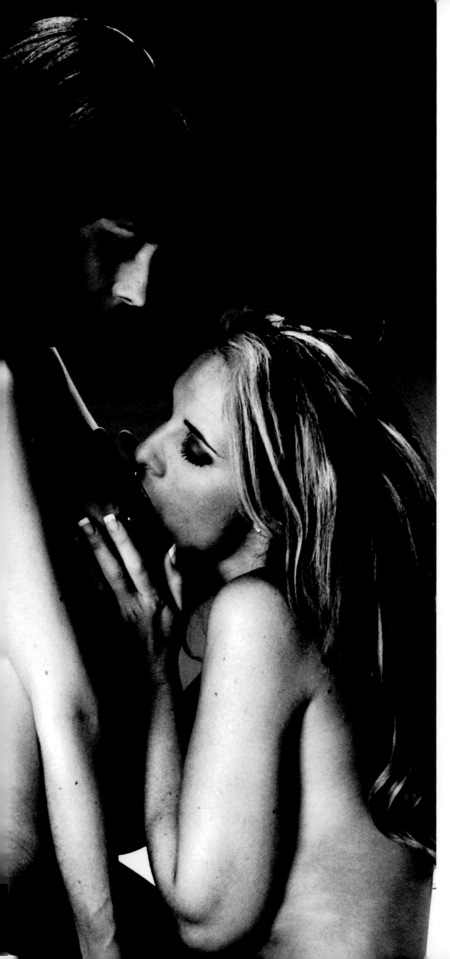

Women vary greatly on the level of stimulation they prefer, so be receptive to a signal, verbal or otherwise, to move on as required. Also a nibble does not equate a bite—biting is dangerous and one should never break another's skin. Be attentive and balance nibbling with other play. Long-term, concentrated stimulation can in fact lead to dulled, or loss of, sensation.

The neck and earlobes are a natural exploration point during a heated make-out session, but venture further and nibble her toes and her inner thighs. Lightly bite her palms and suck on her fingers as you tell her how much you want them inside you.

A great lover can maintain focus and multi-task. Squeeze and nibble on her nipples while fingering her or utilizing a toy to stimulate her lower region. Mix it up by rolling her over and rubbing your pussy up and down her calf and on the heel of her foot as you nibble her sweet buns.

During oral sex, as she grows increasingly wet and swells with desire, try a dainty nibble on her clitoris between tongue flits. A slight tug with the teeth on her labia is also a lustful expression indicating that you're enjoying her so much you're unable to resist nibbling her goods. Don't let her climax stop you. Stay below to explore her inner thighs and hips, even returning to the clitoris until she pushes you away!

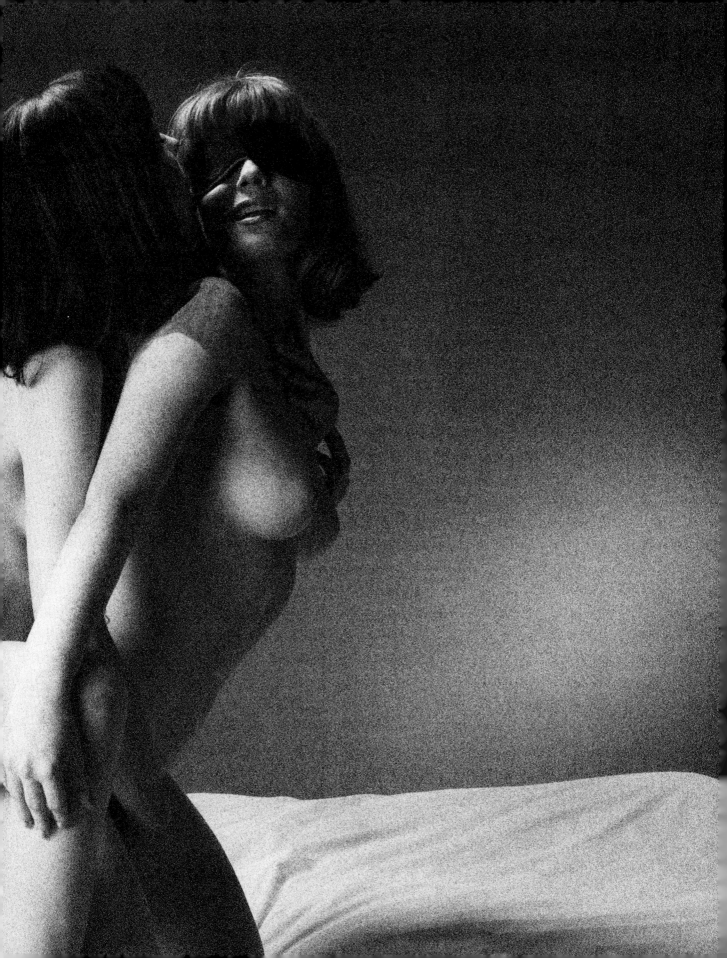

Sexual response is a complex set of many physiological, emotional, and intellectual reactions. The physiological response to behaving naughtily is akin to our natural "fight or flight" reaction to stress, when the adrenal gland secretes adrenaline, a real turn–on.

naughty

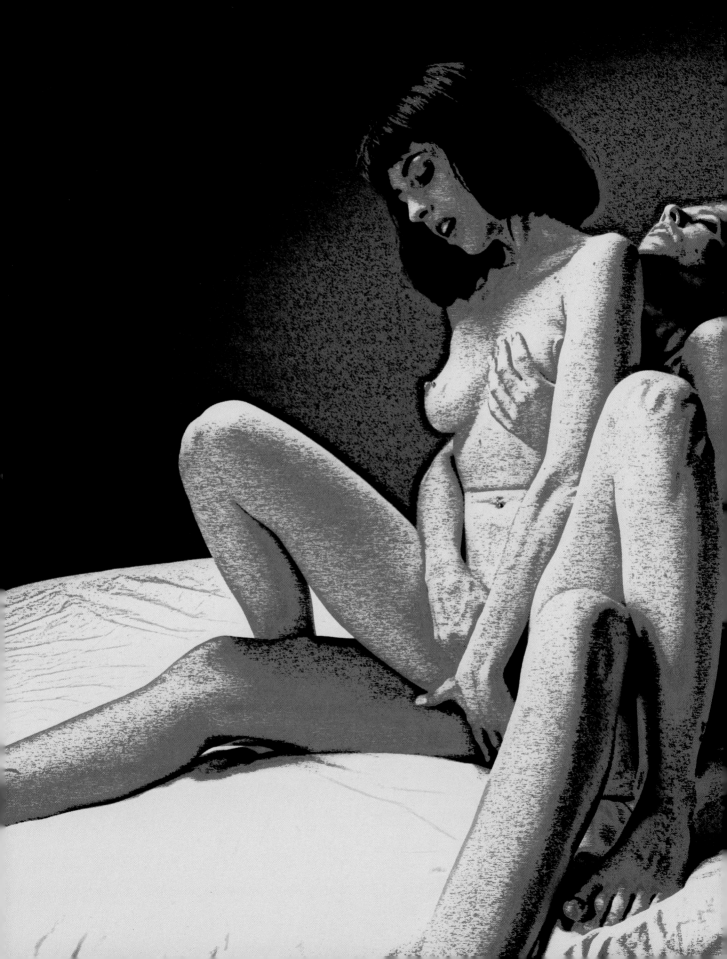

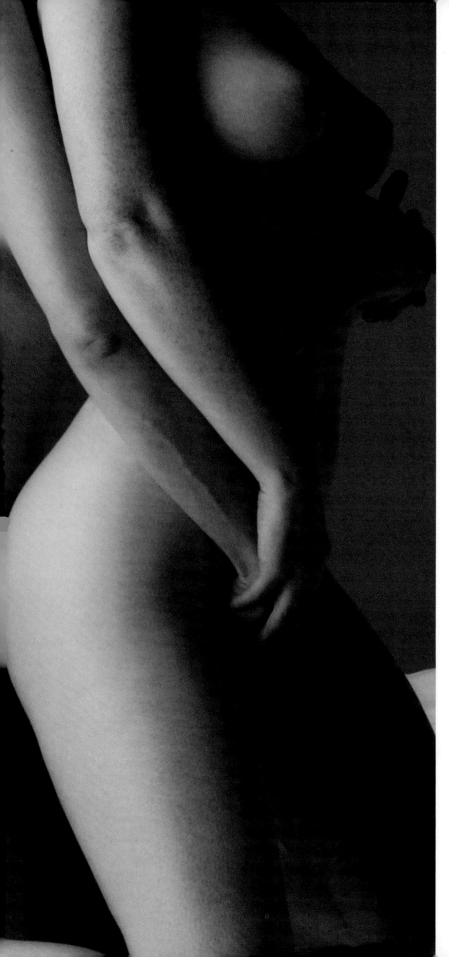

Over time, the meaning of naughty, especially in a sexual context, has evolved into a more lighthearted, mischievous, mildly disobedient, and often suggestive behavior. Perhaps this is the result of the longstanding appeal of the outlaw.

Trespass, disobey, be loud, and get dirty. It's fun to be naughty. Push the envelope, place a racy phone call to your lover, covet a secret, then reveal it to your lover and giggle at your wickedness. For both you and your lover, choosing an unfamiliar "dark" road is thrilling, and being sexually rewarded for behaving naughtily is exhilarating.

What sexual impropriety gets your heart racing by just imagining doing it? Do it. Sit in your favorite chair and read aloud a passage of erotica while masturbating. Let her listen and let her watch. Undress. Turn up the music and dance naked in front of the mirror, you little Jezebel. Is what you desire unspeakable? A bit more radical than your typical pillow talk? Whisper.

Give yourself a climax in the middle of the day, between meetings perhaps. Does you lover have a tough day ahead of her? Slip last night's panties into her briefcase. When she returns home, greet her in the kitchen and seduce her with a lap dance as an appetizer.

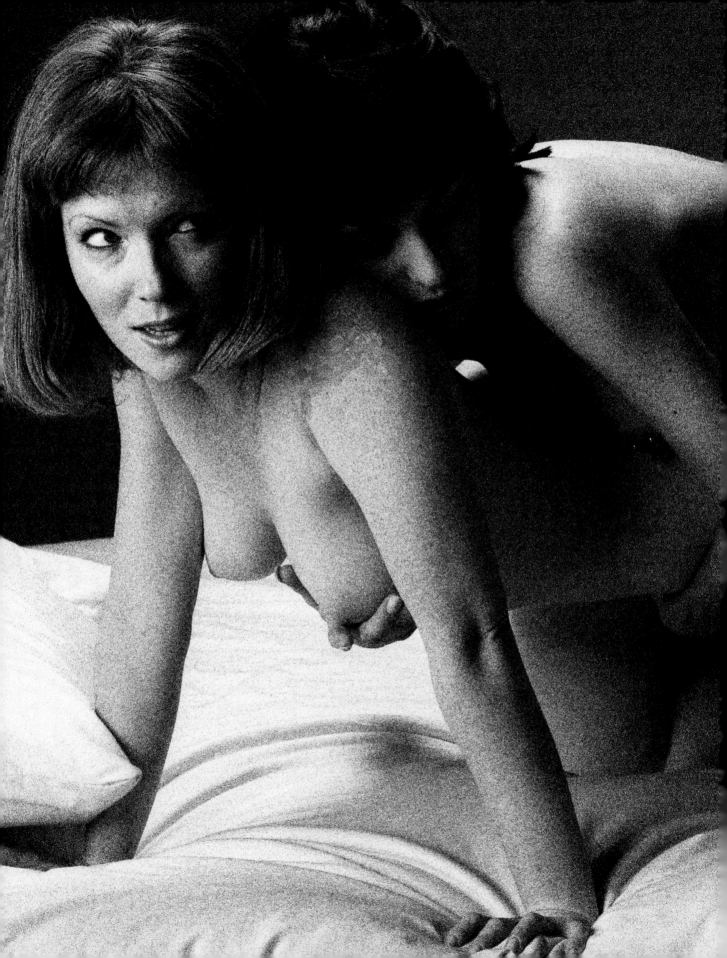

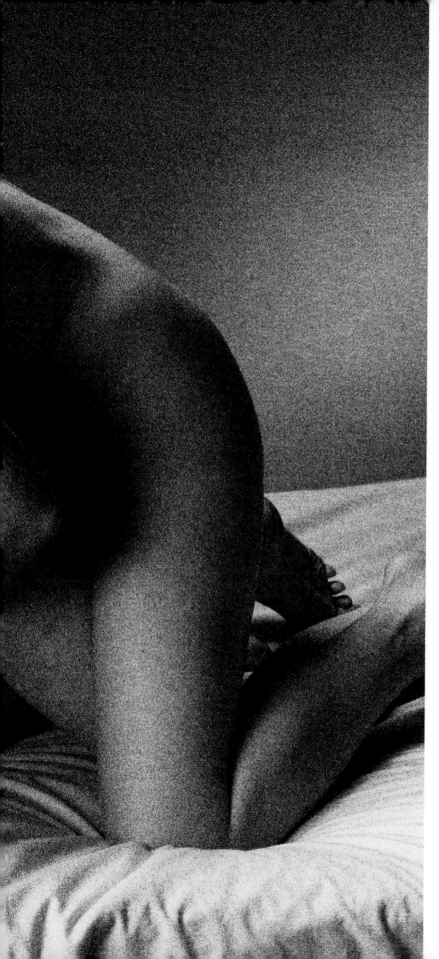

Strap-on a pocket vibrator or "pack" a dildo and wear it to work-out at the gym or for a particularly enjoyable grocery shopping escapade. Because much of the clitoris is located internally, many mistakenly think it's small and that subsequently women are unaware of it much of the time. We know this is not so, and the empowerment brought on by wearing this amusing and sexy "strap-on clit extension" is sure to add a swagger to your step. Celebrate "clitoris awareness day."

Don't save your lingerie for a date or special occasion. Wearing a garter belt or silk panties will make you feel sexy, more confident and powerful the whole day through.

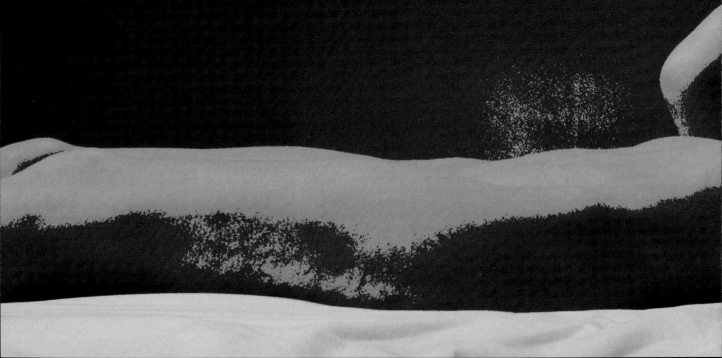

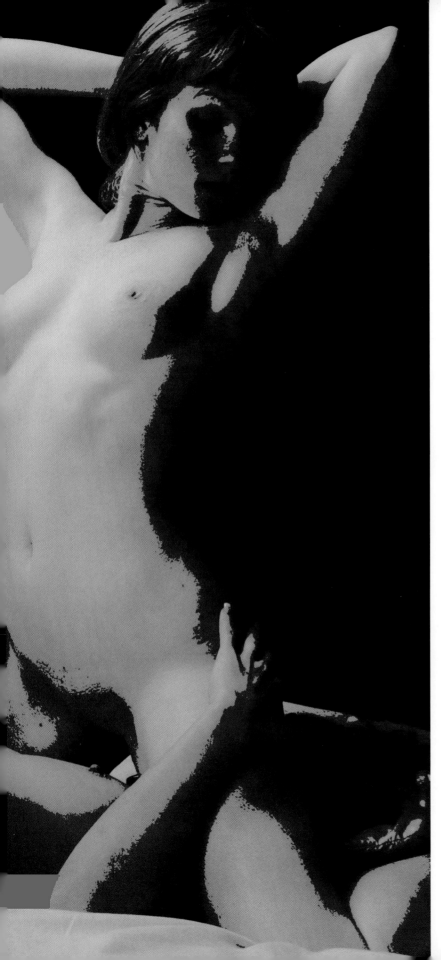

See a blue movie. There are very hot movies out there, some with high production values and more and more being made for women by women. Freeze-frame and mimic a new position or scenario, or just have sex while the film rolls. Making love while a porn movie screens in the background is like attending a sex party without having to deal with the unwanted guests.

Get sexy in a public place. Shopping for a few spring outfits? Fool around in the changing room. Have to work late? When your lover arrives to pick you up, slyly hike up your skirt and shove her under the desk to have her way with you as you wrap up the paperwork or are writing the end of the day e-mail to the boss. Another holiday cocktail party? How about a quickie with your girl on the spare room's coat-check bed. A soft chinchilla against your bare ass is an added treat.

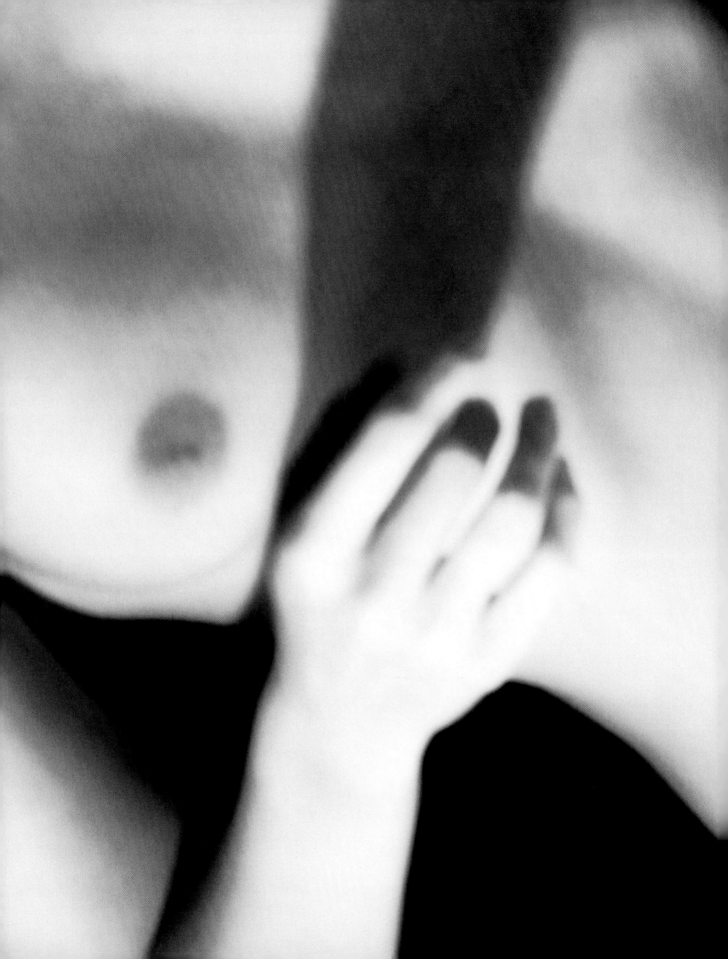

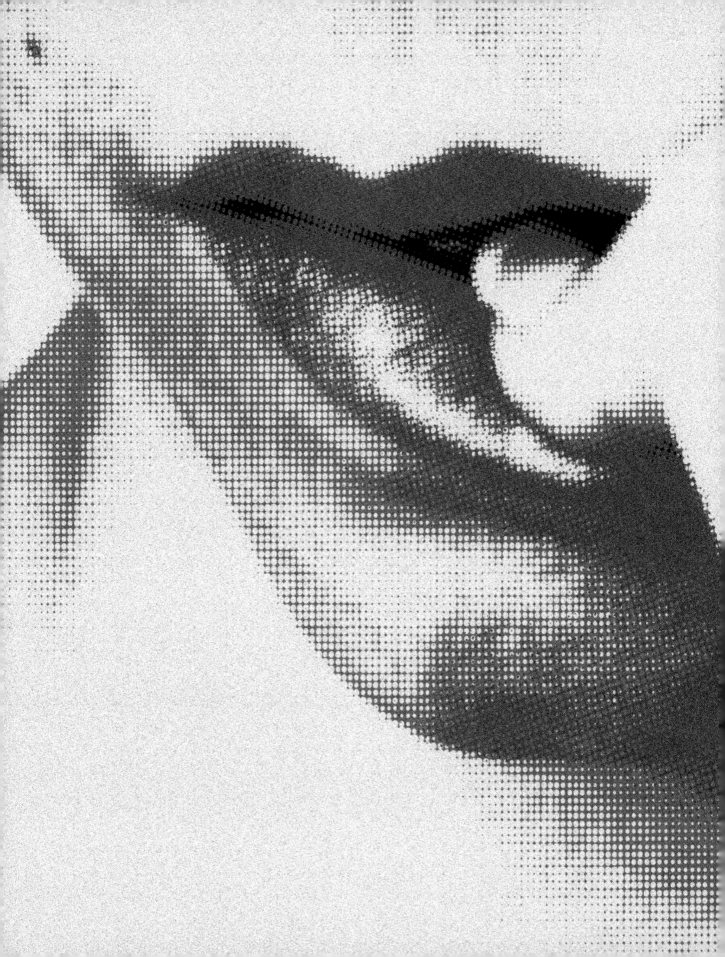

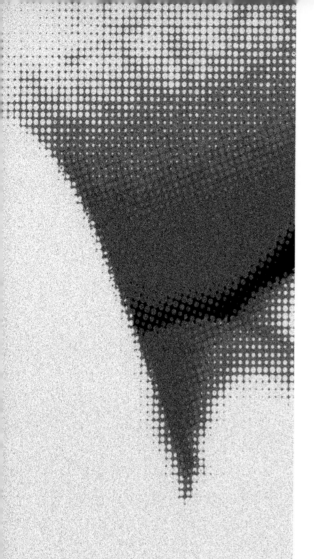

When a woman penetrates another woman, it is generally with her fingers that she first enters to feel the wet warmth of her lover. What an amazing gift, to gain admittance and feel her body respond from this entirely intimate perspective.

fingers

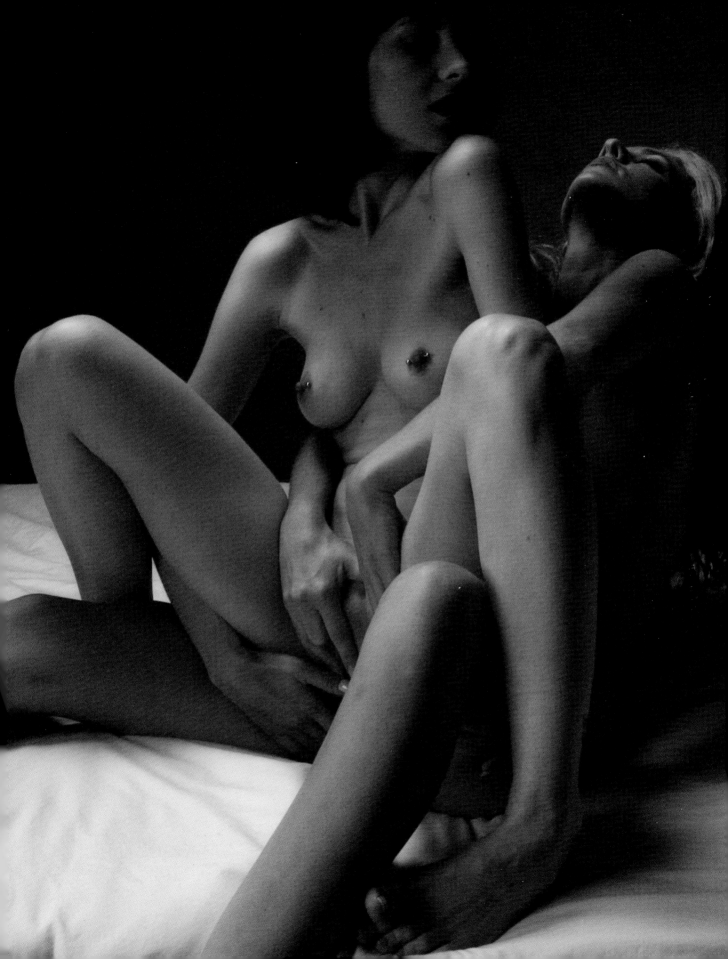

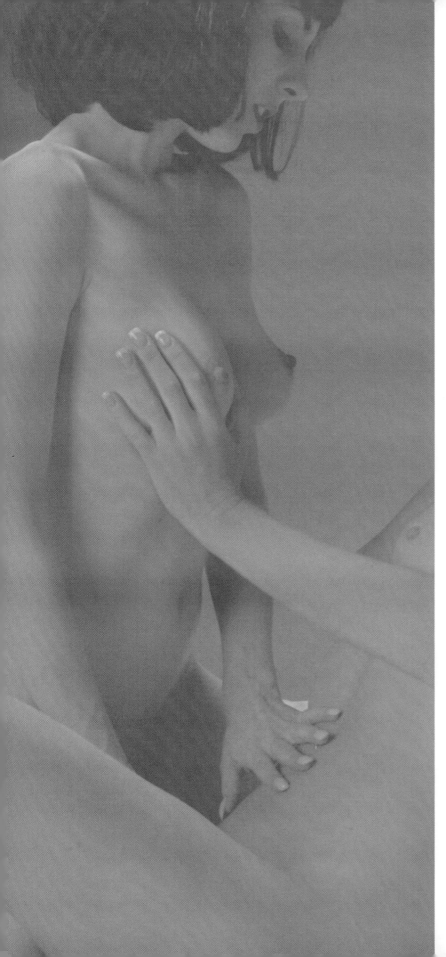

Despite all the wonderful toys now available to lesbians, these natural, strong digits called fingers are still a favorite tool for many. Fingers can travel everywhere, roaming across her entire body, tugging at clothing, tweaking her nipples, pressing, fondling, pulling, rubbing, feeling her all over.

Lesbians slyly study women's fingers. Hands tell a lot about a person. Imagine the intimate, private, and luxurious places they could travel on your body. A casual touch on the hand can be especially intimate and communicate volumes to someone in whom you are interested.

Penetrate her slowly at first, and insert one finger, then two. Put these fingers in your mouth to taste her and perhaps to moisten your fingers before reinserting, especially if she's still tight and not very wet yet, then slide back inside. Three fingers and then four, an achievement otherwise known as a "Whole in One." With your free hand touch yourself to feel how your pussy is responding to your increased arousal. As your fingers slide in and out of her vagina, use your other hand or your mouth to simultaneously stimulate the clitoris. Our fingertips are full of nerve receptors, so when our fingers are touching, rubbing, probing or being kissed, nibbled or sucked, the sexual sensations are certainly mutual.

Finger her pussy while one or both of you are standing, either facing one another or with one lover pressed against the other's backside. Raise one leg, perhaps draping it over your lover's shoulder for easier access so that her fingers can thrust hard and deep inside at a comfortable angle for her hand and your pussy.

Pamper your hands and hers. Treat her to a hand massage as you lie in bed, stroking each finger and kneading and caressing her palms. Make a date to meet for manicures. Subtly flirt with her while in the salon, letting her know that you are imagining and anticipating her lovely fingers on and in your body.

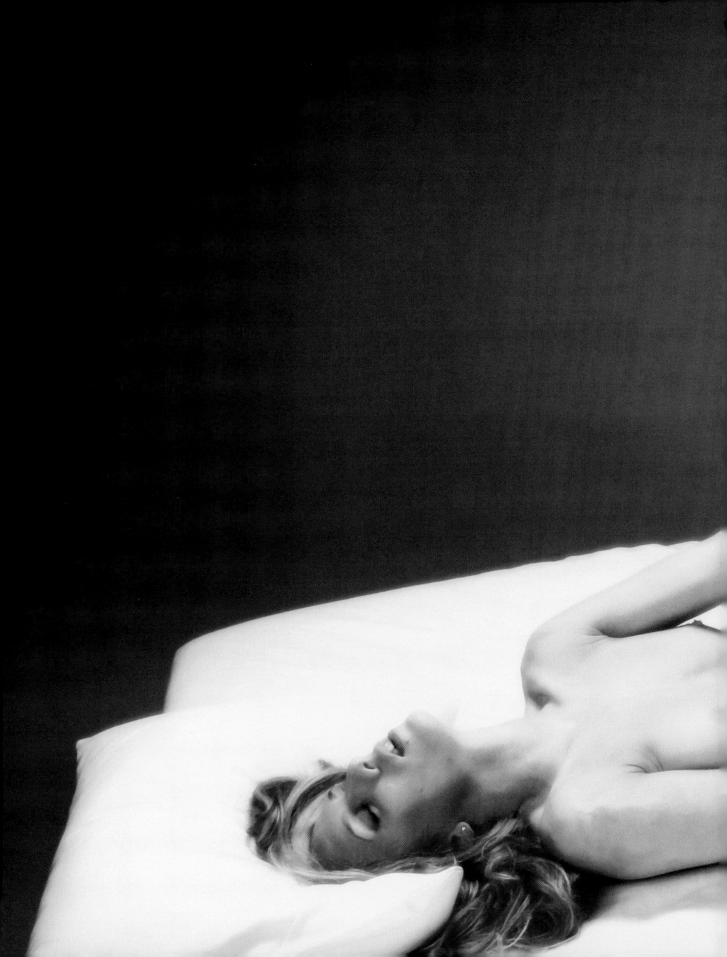

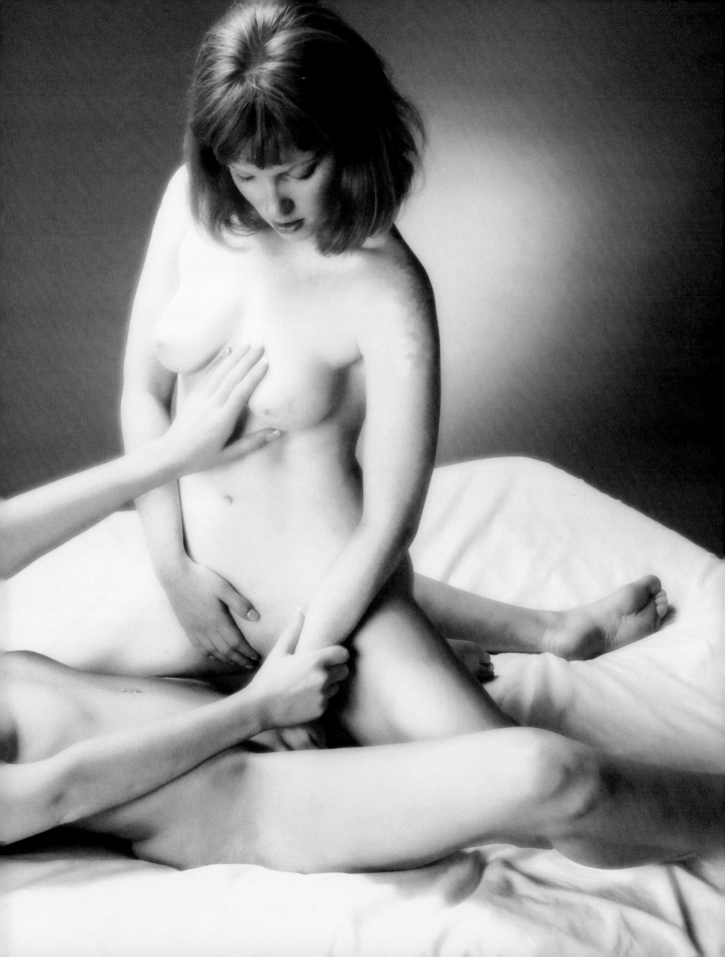

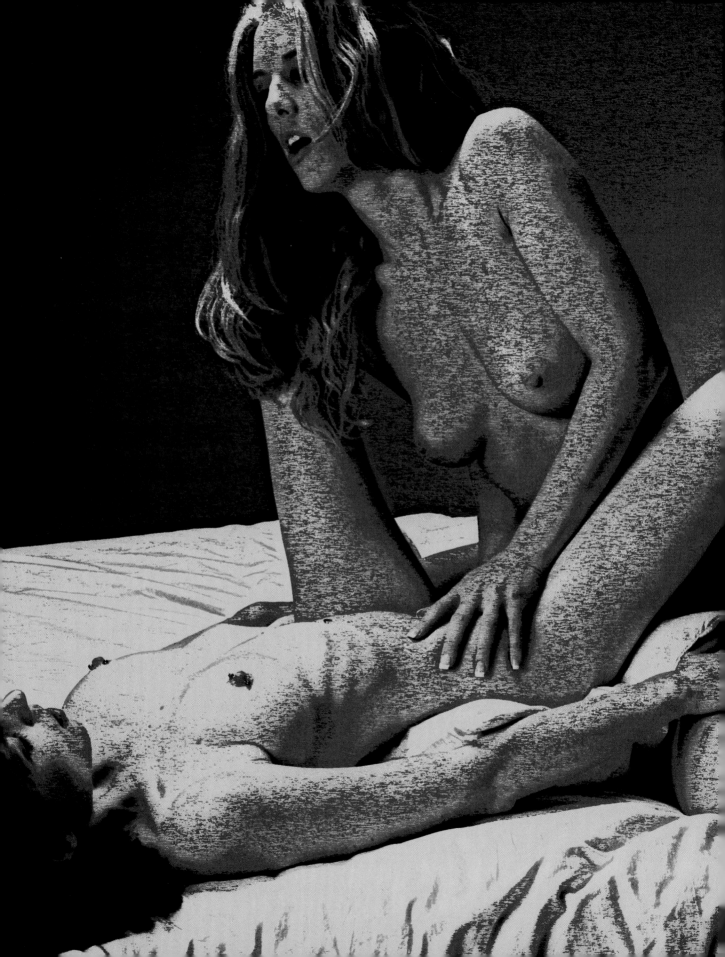

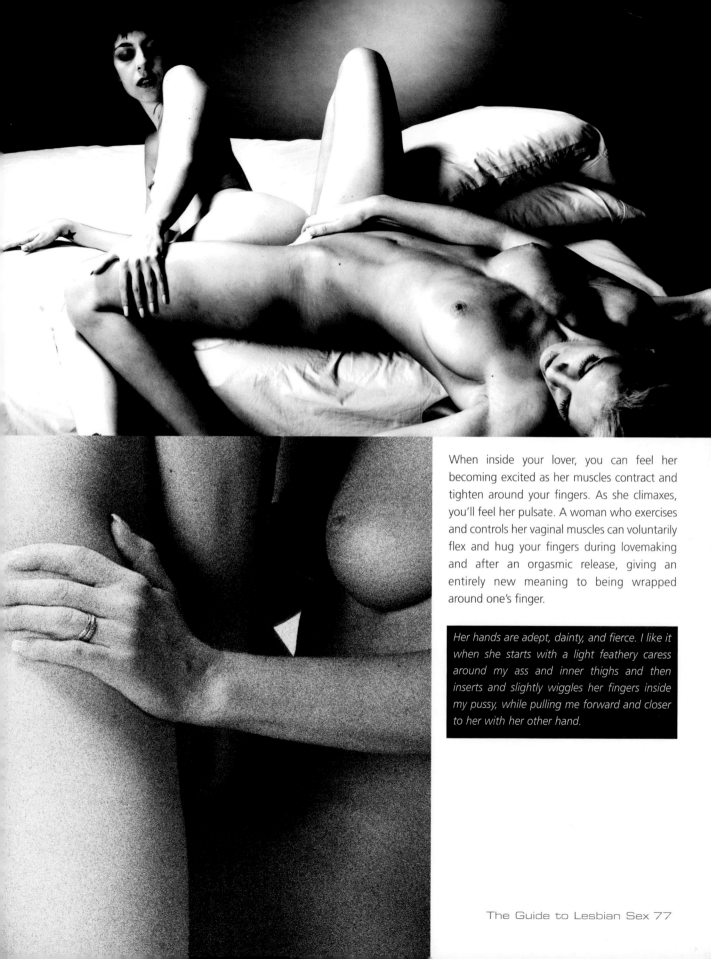

When inside your lover, you can feel her becoming excited as her muscles contract and tighten around your fingers. As she climaxes, you'll feel her pulsate. A woman who exercises and controls her vaginal muscles can voluntarily flex and hug your fingers during lovemaking and after an orgasmic release, giving an entirely new meaning to being wrapped around one's finger.

Her hands are adept, dainty, and fierce. I like it when she starts with a light feathery caress around my ass and inner thighs and then inserts and slightly wiggles her fingers inside my pussy, while pulling me forward and closer to her with her other hand.

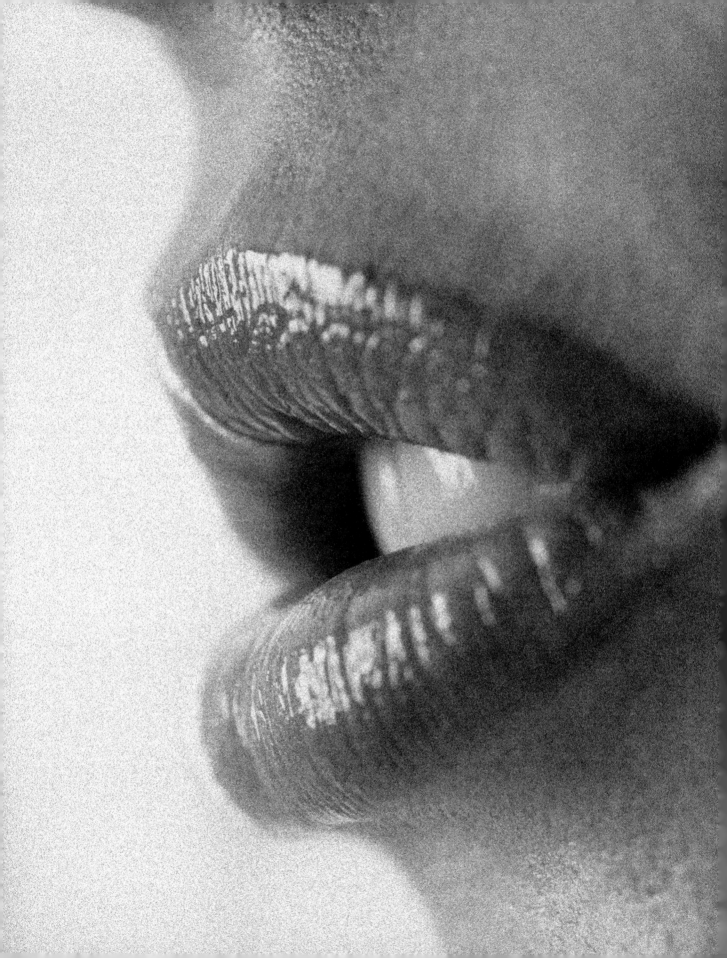

Lips are arguably the sexiest bits of soft tissue on the body. They are incredibly delicate and endlessly expressive. Without lips we would be hard-pressed to flash a pretty smile, speak, pout, or pucker up to kiss.

lips

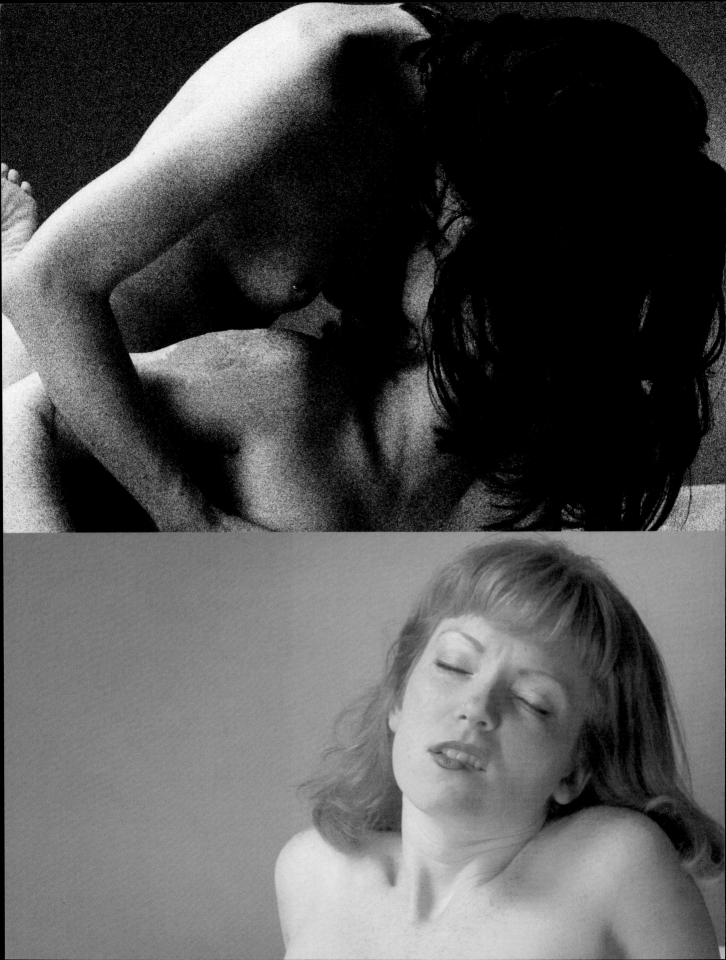

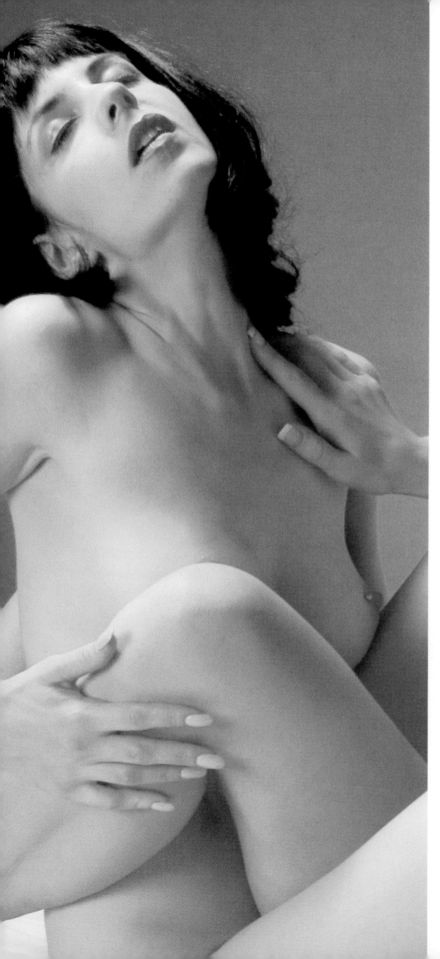

Consumers spend exorbitantly to adorn and enhance their lips. Many women strive for fullness, some by injecting foreign substances and others by utilizing topical products that contain stimulating ingredients such as cinnamon, peppermint, caffeine, or niacin, which aggravate the lips in varying degrees, increasing blood flow and causing lips to swell and redden. This cosmetic trend is perhaps a link to our powerful subconscious as plump lips resemble an aroused vagina. The lips of the labia are in turn often said to emulate the petals of flowers, held to be among the most exquisite gifts of natural beauty on Earth.

Few lips are a perfect pair. Just as one breast tends to be bigger than the other, the mouth's bottom lip is most often larger than the top, and one labia is usually longer or more voluptuous than its counterpart. Labia swell and sometimes change in color when a woman is sexually aroused.

Moistness implies sexual health, so it follows that the glistening of a pearly white lip gloss will encourage the imagination to wander into the world of wetness. Lick your lips. It's sexy to watch a woman whom you desire lick her lips. Imagine her lips touching yours. Imagine her soft, wet lips exploring your body.

Women also choose to enhance their lips by applying a flattering color to suit a particular environment or event, a mood or an intention. Accentuation is taken a step further by lining the lips with a colored pencil. Red lips imply power, a softer rose hue is romantic, and *au natural* balms signify a confident, no-frills woman who nonetheless recognizes the value of softness.

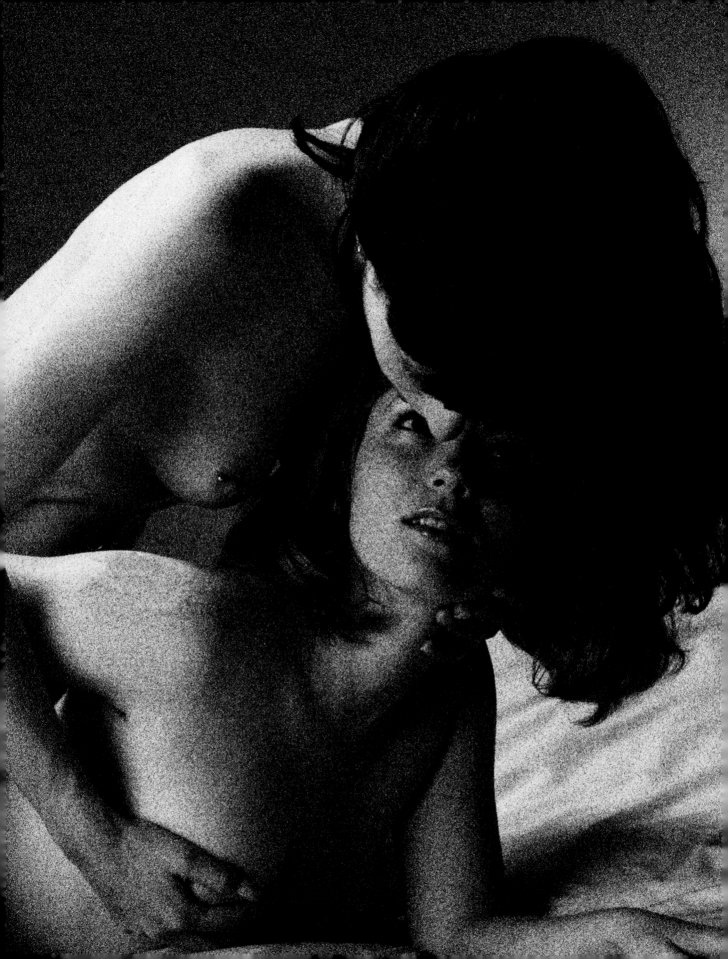

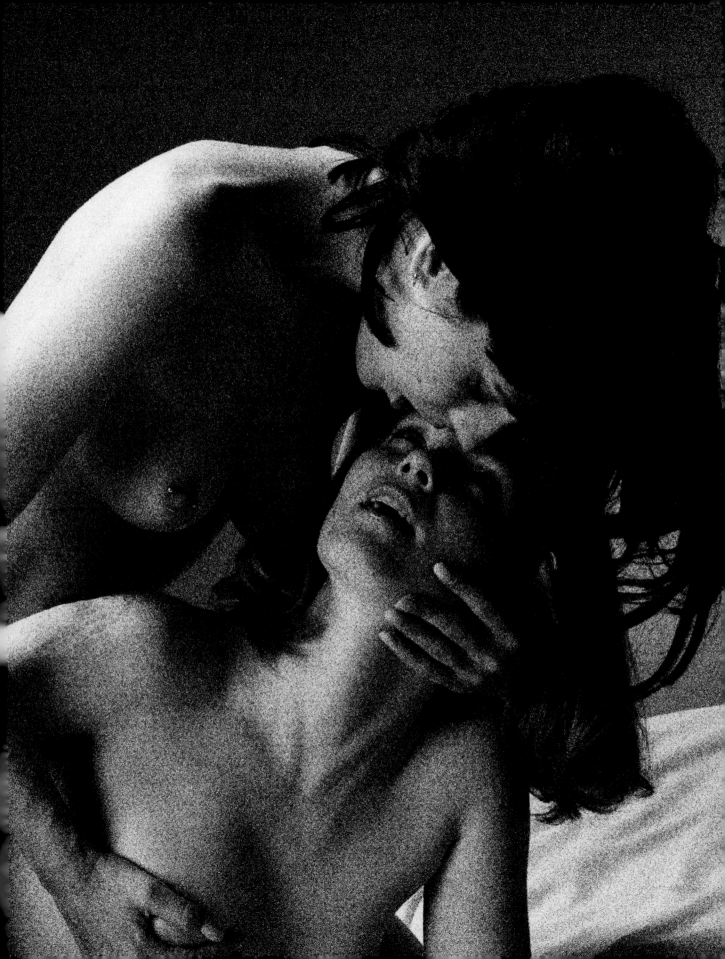

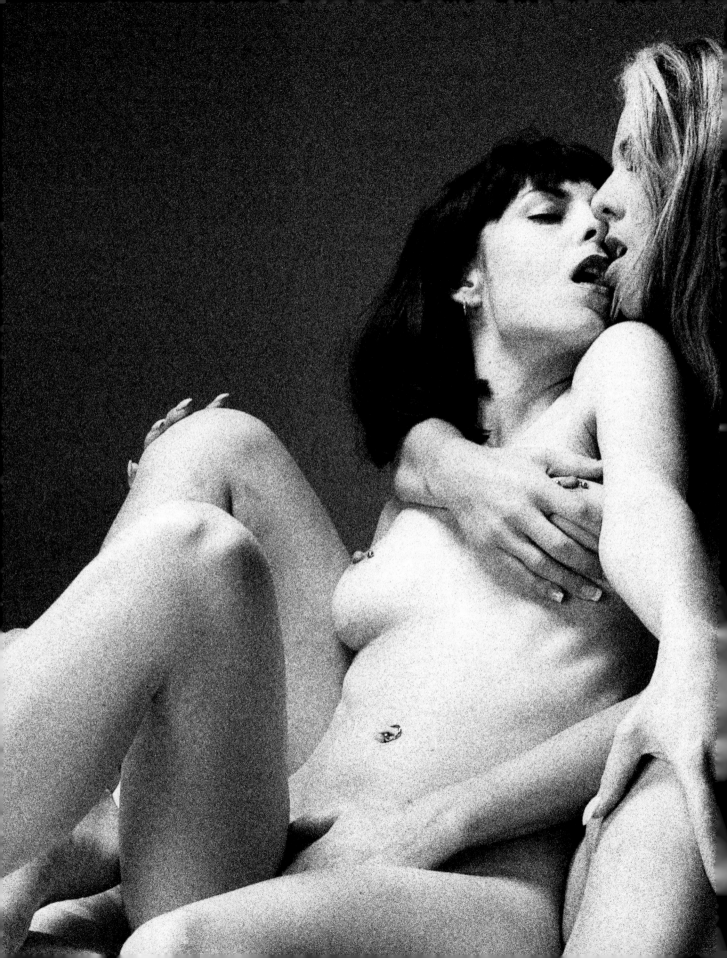

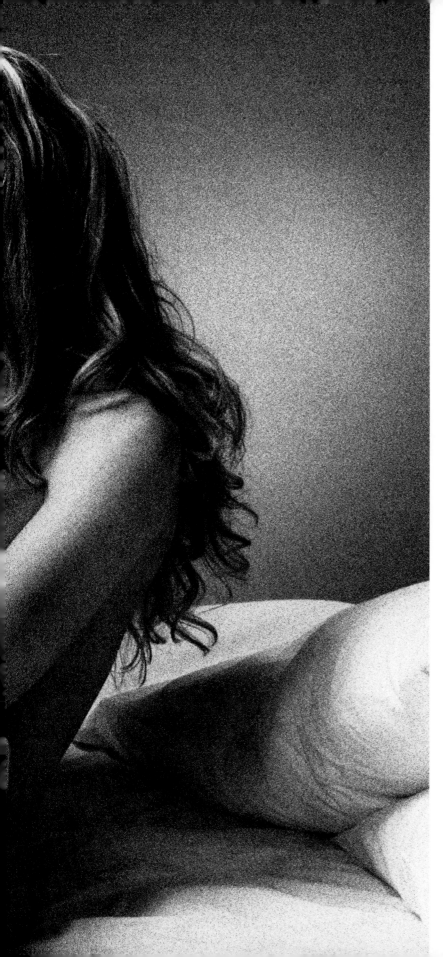

Virtually worldwide, a kiss is recognized as both a greeting and a sign of affection. The beginning of a courtship is often sealed with an intimate kiss, but interestingly, so is the end of a relationship. Kisses can be blown, softly pecked, a lingering, firm lip-to-lip press or open-mouthed, tongue twirling expressions of desire.

Lips deserve the extra attention they implore. Try slow and soft nibbles, beginning on her lower lip. She'll tingle with anticipation when you spend some time emulating on her sensitive mouth just how you plan to eat her pussy.

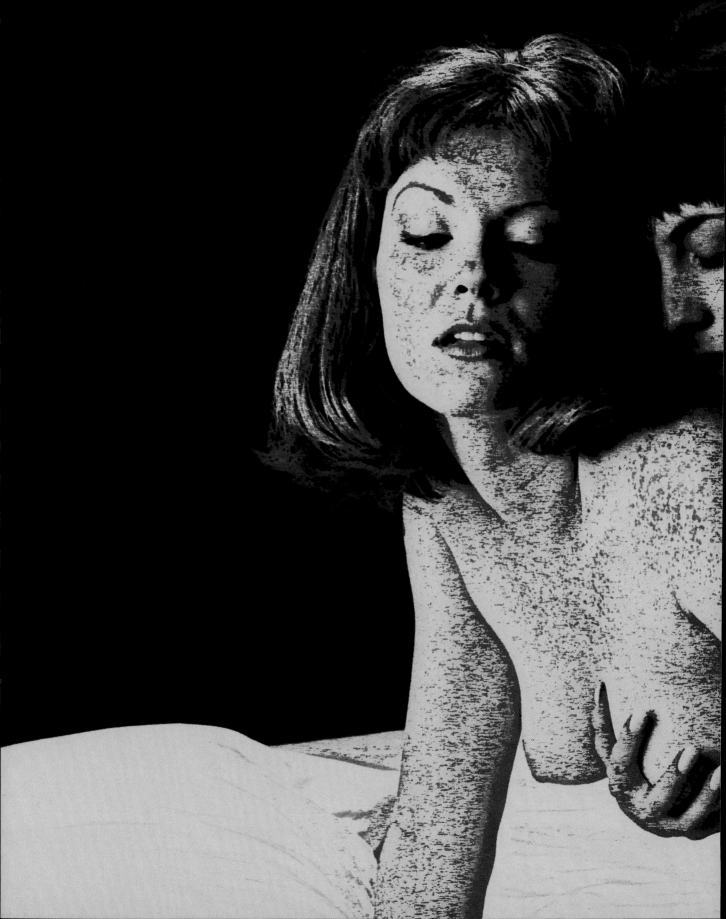

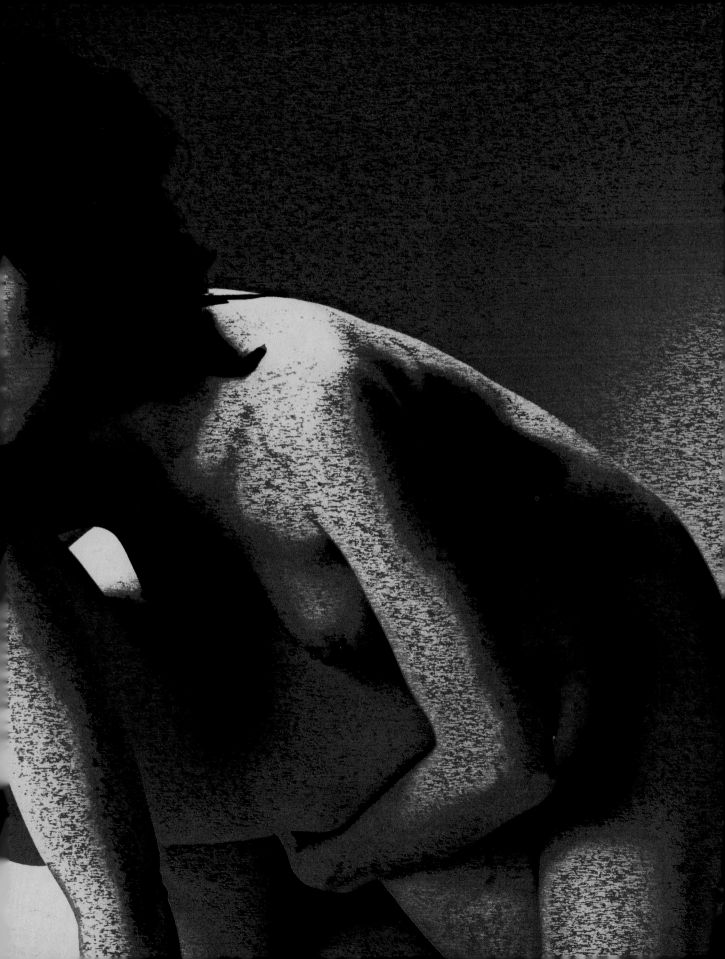

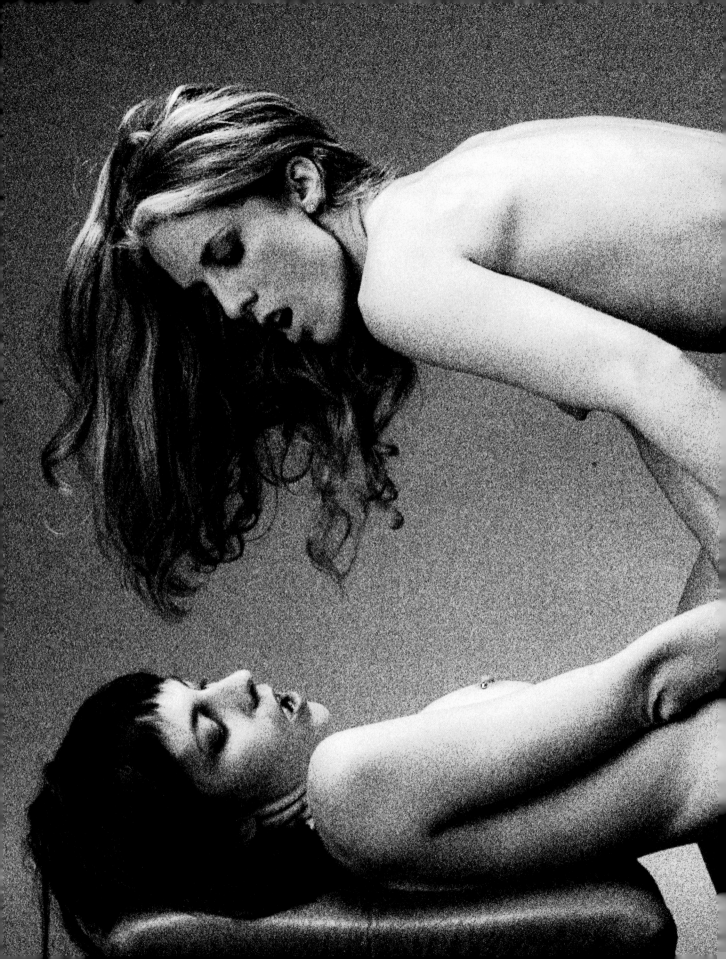

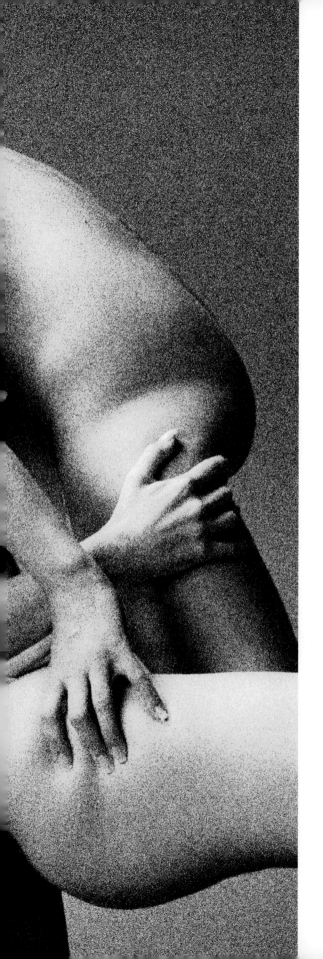

Effective communication is the basis for developing and maintaining a connection with another person. We share our most intimate thoughts, ideas, and desires with our lovers because we enjoy expressing ourselves and we seek affirmation for, and reinforcement of, the choices we make throughout our lives.

tell

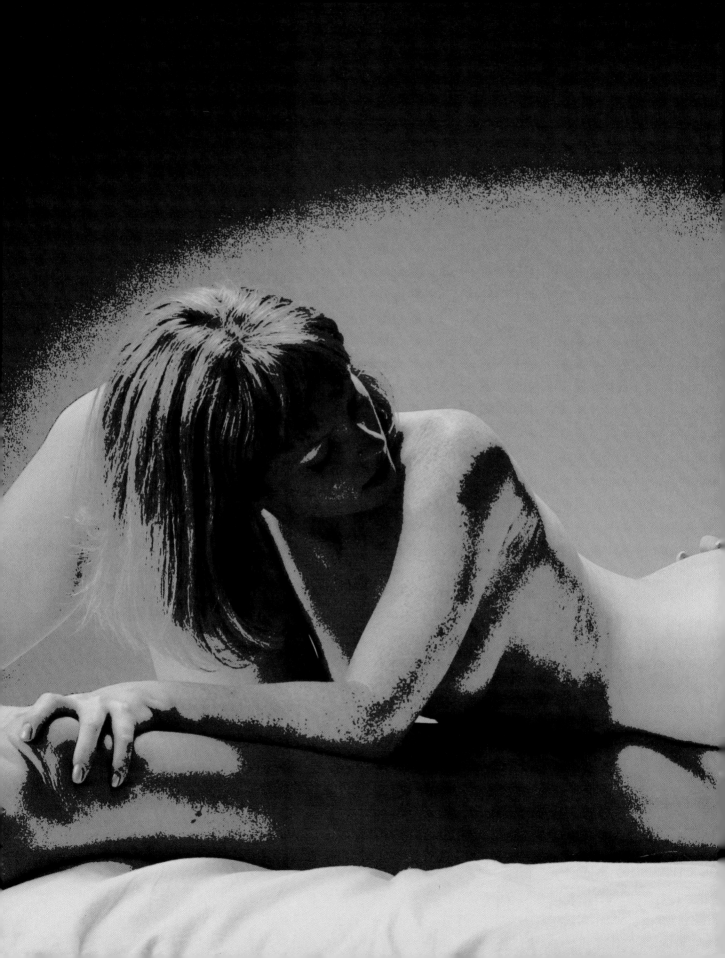

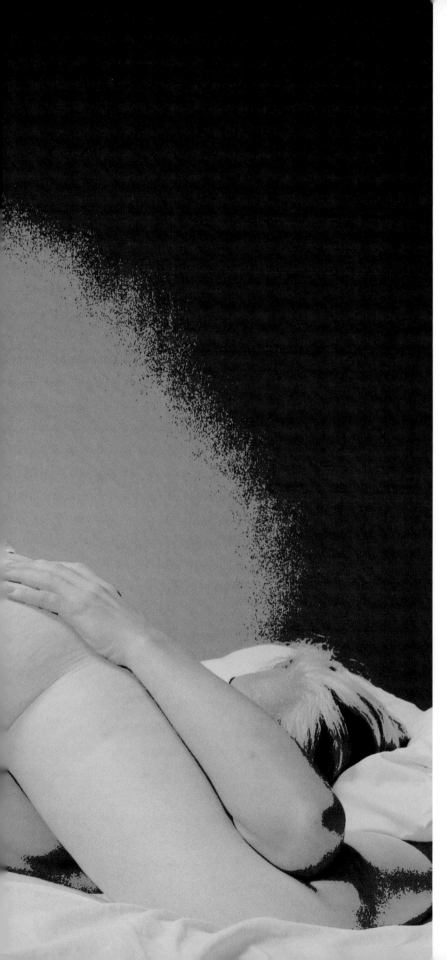

Boundaries change over time and as a relationship deepens. One woman may become more open with regard to sex, whether this involves frequency, the level of intimacy, varying sexual positions, or experimentation. Another woman may have been more willing to experiment in her youth but is a bit more inhibited today. Communicate to one another changes in boundaries and desires at all stages of a relationship. For lovers to stay in love, mutual candor, privacy, and dignity are essential.

Intimacy increases our level of vulnerability. Sharing is more difficult for some women, especially in this world where there is still judgment, and a lack of global acceptance regarding sexual identity. Consider what is private to you and ponder the value of sharing it with your partner. As often as our hearts and heads sometimes collide, both can also show us the way to enrichment by sharing our deepest desires with others.

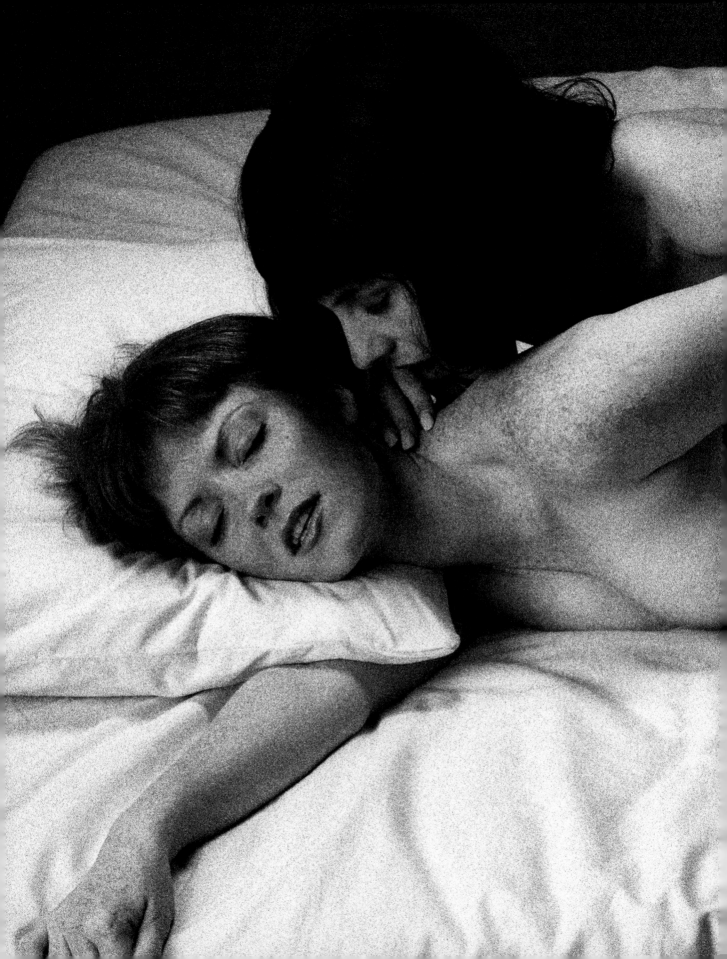

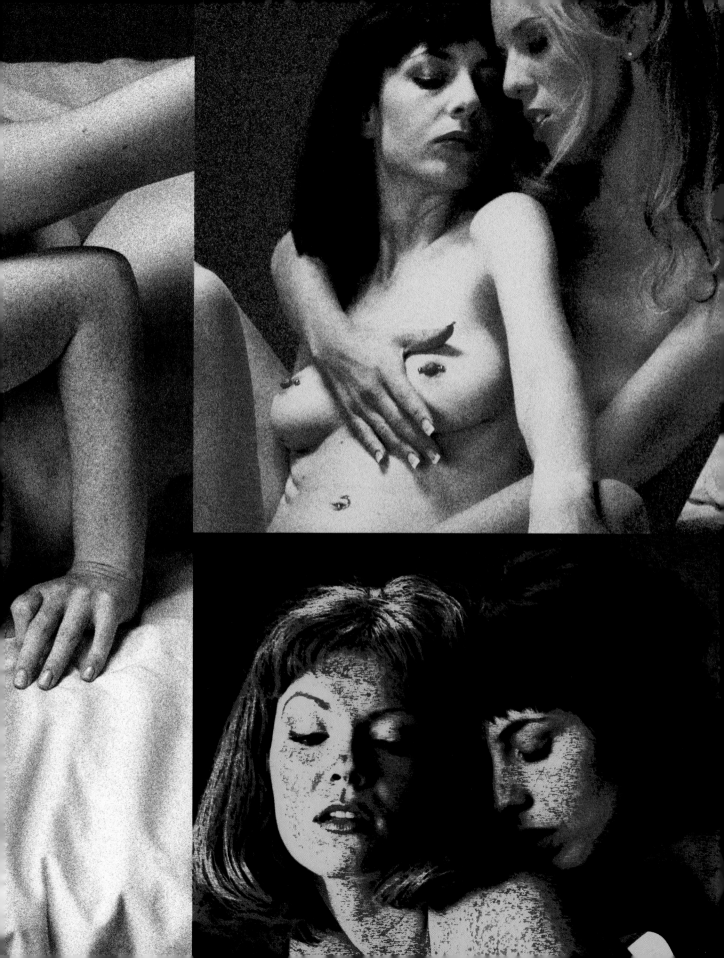

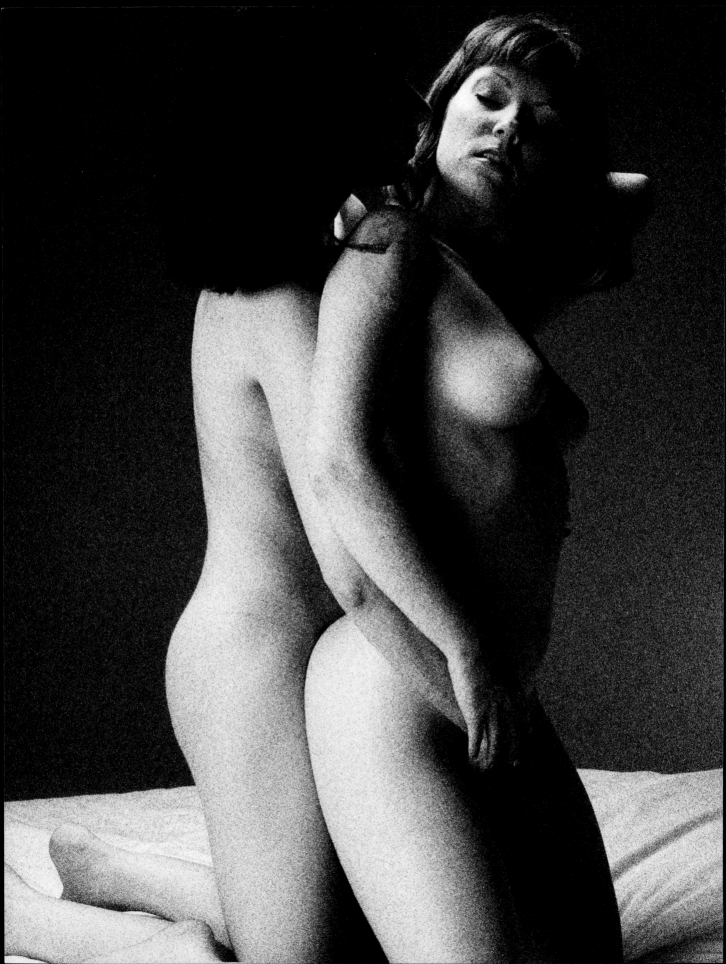

Without "listen," "tell" is of little importance. Communication is a joint effort. As we get to know one another, further defining each other's personality, it is easiest to note the similarities like enjoying the same joke or preferring a particular genre of movie or book, but it is equally important to embrace and encourage our differences. These differences provide the challenges and opportunities that allow us to grow.

Even for two women who have known one another for a while, it remains necessary to articulate each other's desires. You cannot will her tongue to press harder on your clit. Somehow, you have to tell her. Say, "harder" and press her head into you, gently but insistently.

Tell her you like what she's doing to you while she's doing it. Tell her if she's too far to the left. Guide her hand. Moan, groan, sigh and cry out. Tell her you want her to sit on your face. Tell her she has a beautiful body and you would like her to hold it against you. Laugh. Tell her a secret. Tell her she's beautiful. Catch her eye, wink and smile. Every day, tell her that you love her.

A fulfilling sexual relationship revolves around the discovery of what you both want and the conveyance of these assorted desires. Don't be shy. Invite her in.

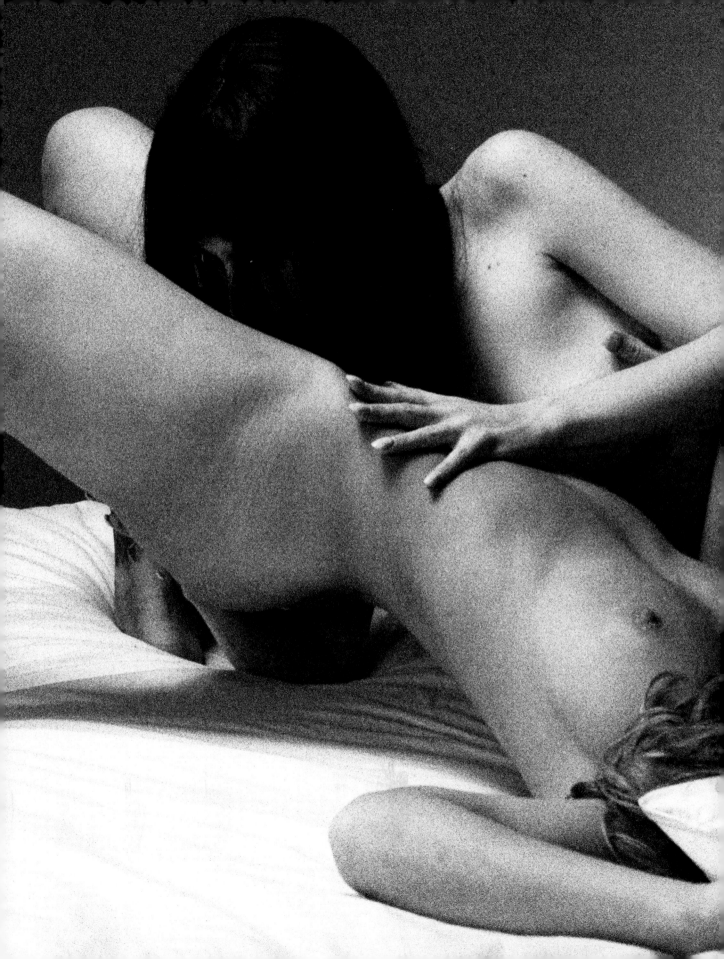

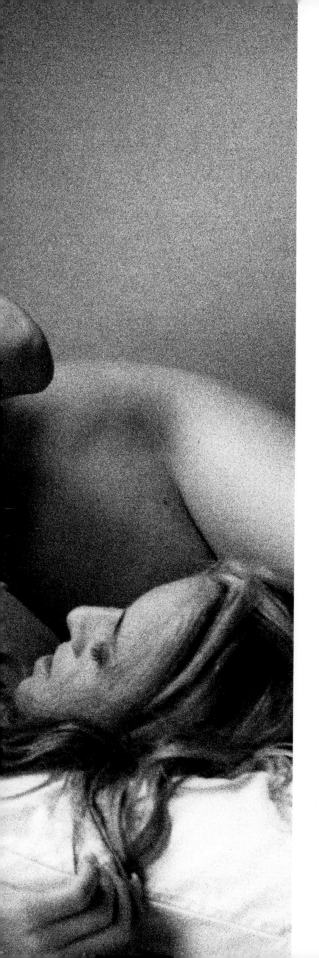

To lick is to pass our tongue along a surface. The tongue is a large bundle of muscles covered with thousands of highly sensitive taste buds and papillae capable of inducing our sexual appetite and enhancing sexual pleasure. It's versatile, pliable, moist, and an ideal texture for sex. While other animals are practical with their licking, incorporating it into their hygiene regimen and licking another to express affection, humans tend to lick either as a part of eating or as an erotic activity.

lick

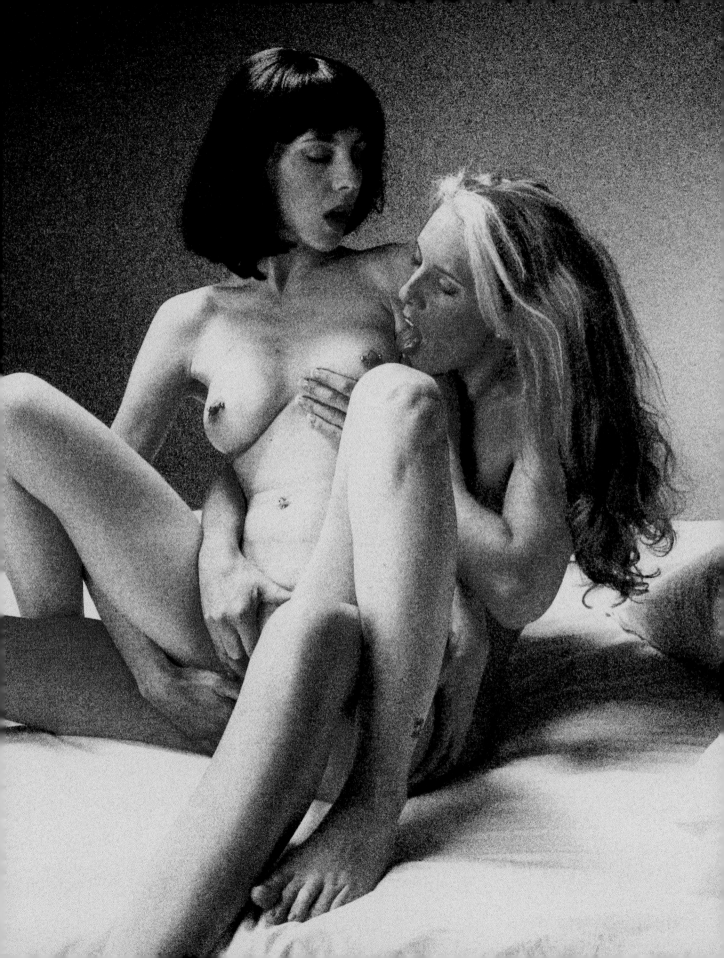

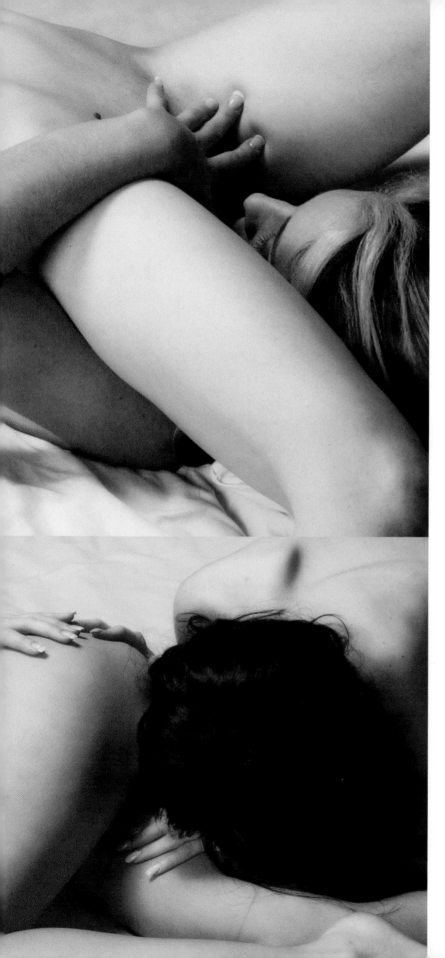

There is so much to lick — ice cream, ripe fruit, and every nook and cranny of the female body. A finger can be licked to make it less slippery, like when flipping pages of a book, or to make it more wet when behaving sensually.

Individuals will exhibit varying styles of licking. Some women are very free and enthusiastic, while others prefer more delicate and controlled licking. Assuming she is genetically predisposed, a woman might first curl her tongue into a conical shape before plunging in to explore her lover's pussy. Licks can be flits of the ultra-sensitive tip of the tongue or can probe deep.

Courting and pleasing the pussy need not be overwhelming or perplexing. Let's break down the sexual act of cunnilingus, a deeply personal expression of passion, into useful tips and techniques that are sure to enhance your muffdiving skills lickety–split!

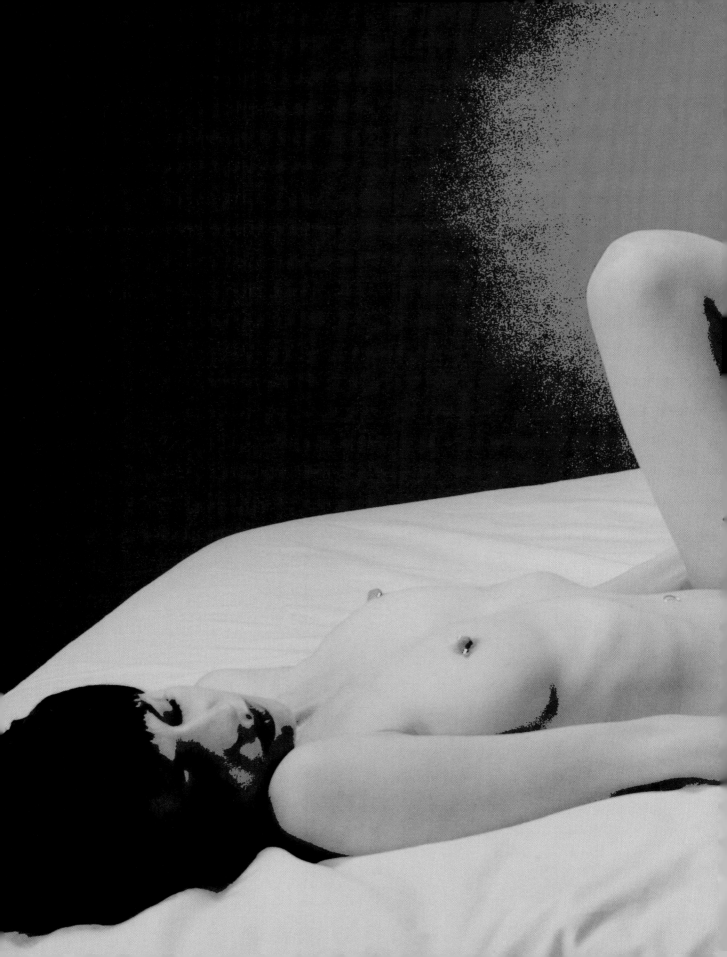

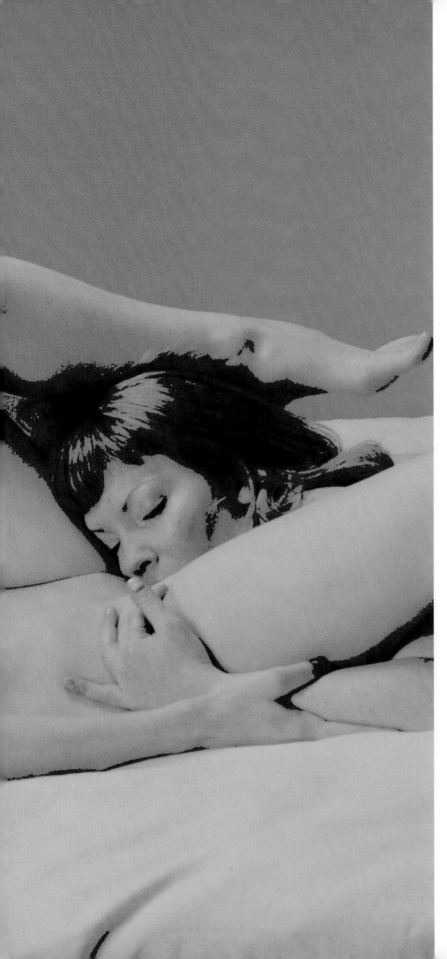

If she's still wearing panties, warm her with a huff and a puff through the fabric, a sexy sensation prior to the panties being peeled off in the heat of passionate foreplay. Then indulge her with slow, broad licks on the lips of her outer labia, perineum, and hood. Take time to discover the textures, valleys, and peeks of her lovely pussy.

Make your way to her inner labia, exploring the folds, then move up under the glans or hood to tease the hardening clitoris. Let your tongue dive into her moist, warm vaginal opening. Repeat this, falling into a rhythm of intermittent licks and dives. Take her entire pussy into your mouth. Lightly nibble and taste her. Show her how much you love to eat her pussy.

As you feel her clitoris hardening, her vulva swelling and her vagina moistening and opening to welcome you, begin more focused stimulation. Solicit and gauge her responses and adjust position, the direction of the movement and the pressure accordingly. It's okay to ask her, "do you like that?"

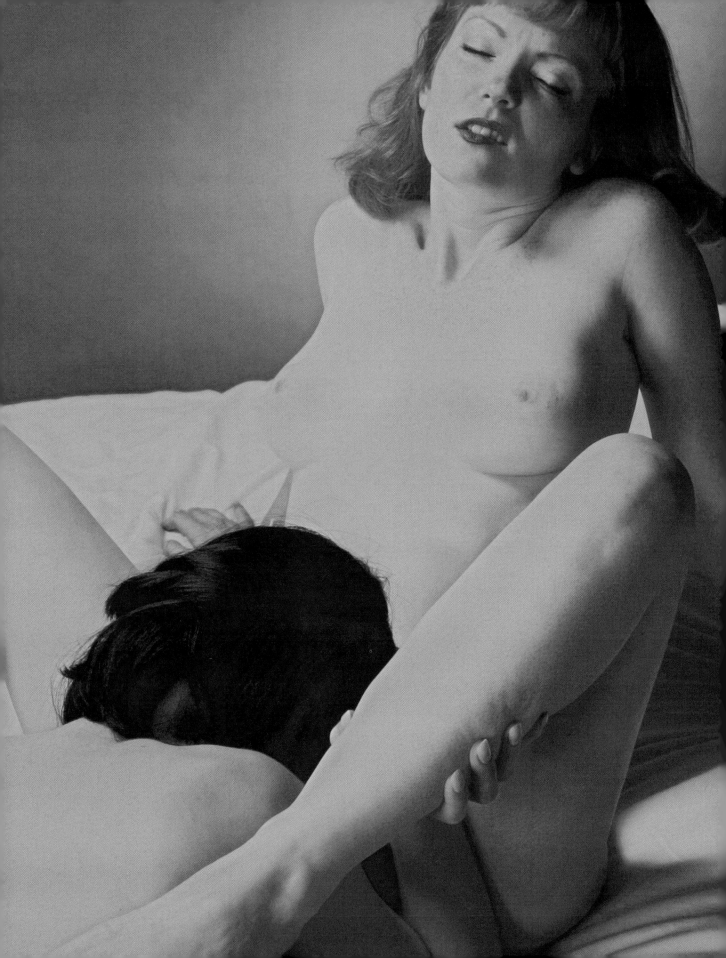

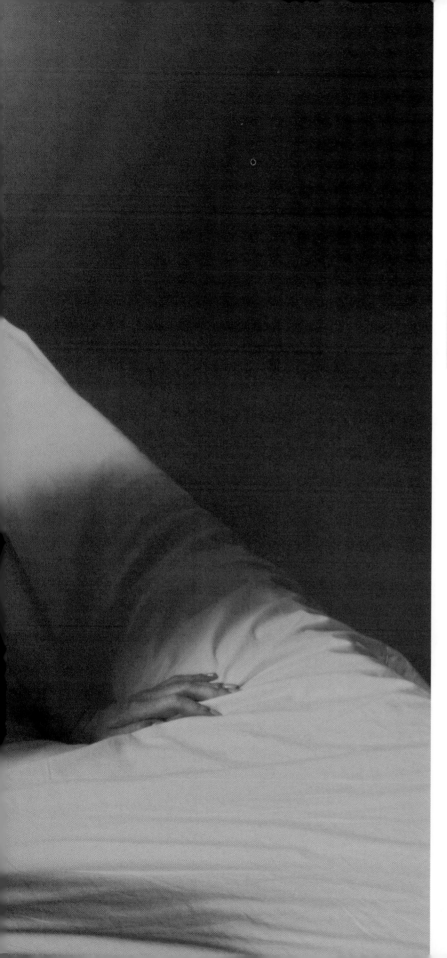

To bring her to a climax, return your concentration to the swelling tip of her clitoris while your fingers continue to work in tandem with your mouth. Fingers can assist the tongue on the clitoris, slide in and out of the vagina or reach up to stroke her breast and tug on a nipple. Variation is fun but if the rhythm and level of pressure are working, stick to the beat. Repetition, endurance, focus, and patience are integral to experiencing the most superb, orally-induced orgasm.

My heart's racing as I feel her tongue tickle the curve of my ass and explore my inner thighs. She rolls me on my back and promptly dives into my sweet spot. I tense up, touch the top of her head and ask her to slow down so I can feel her tongue inside me.

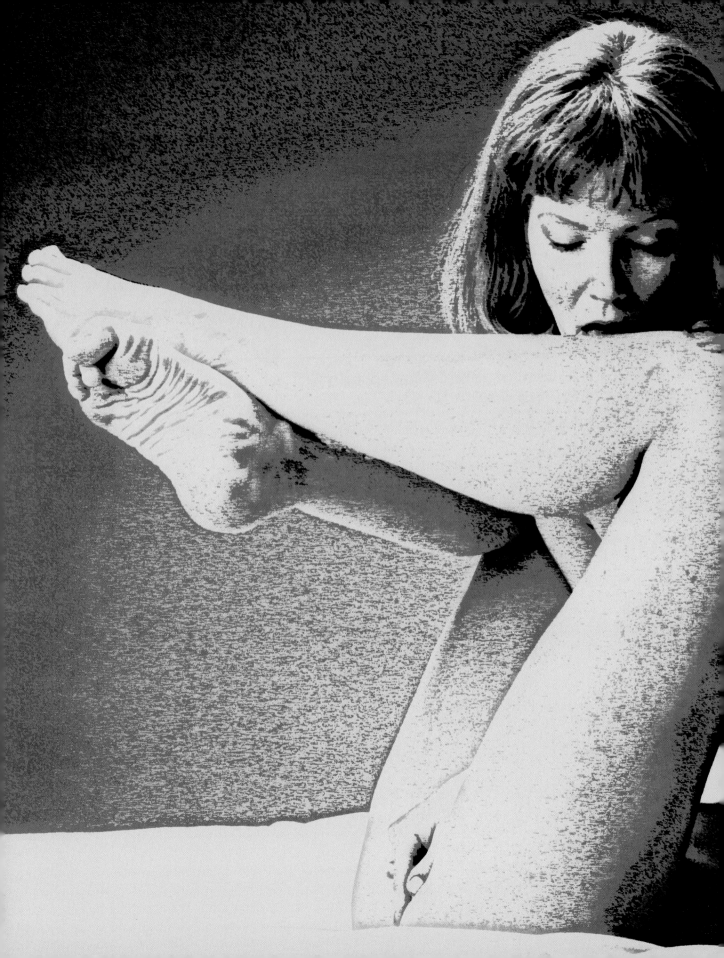

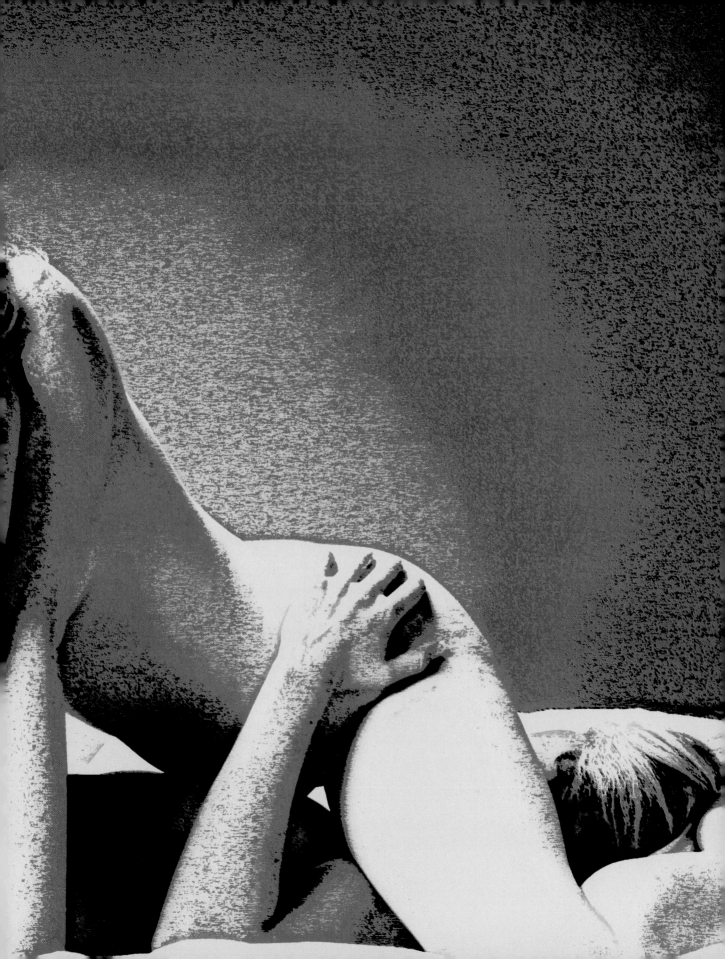

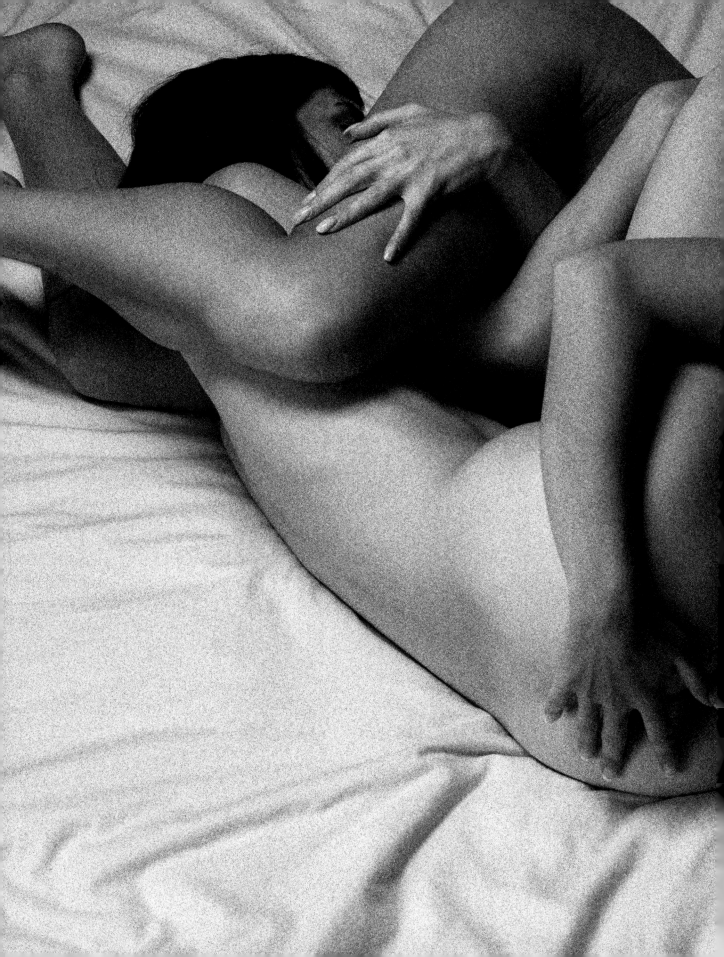

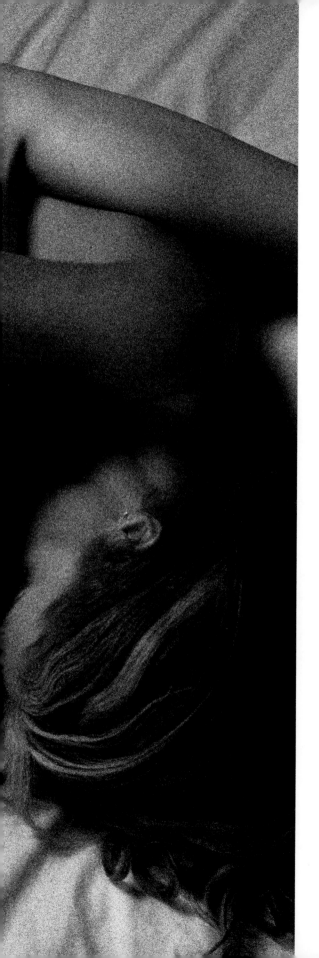

To taste is to distinguish the flavor, sensation, and quality of whatever we take into our mouths. If we respond positively to what we taste, it in fact drives our hunger and increases our appetite. Having taste also defines one's sophistication level, and can refer to a personal preference, such as having a taste for fresh figs with goat cheese or for sex with the lights on.

taste

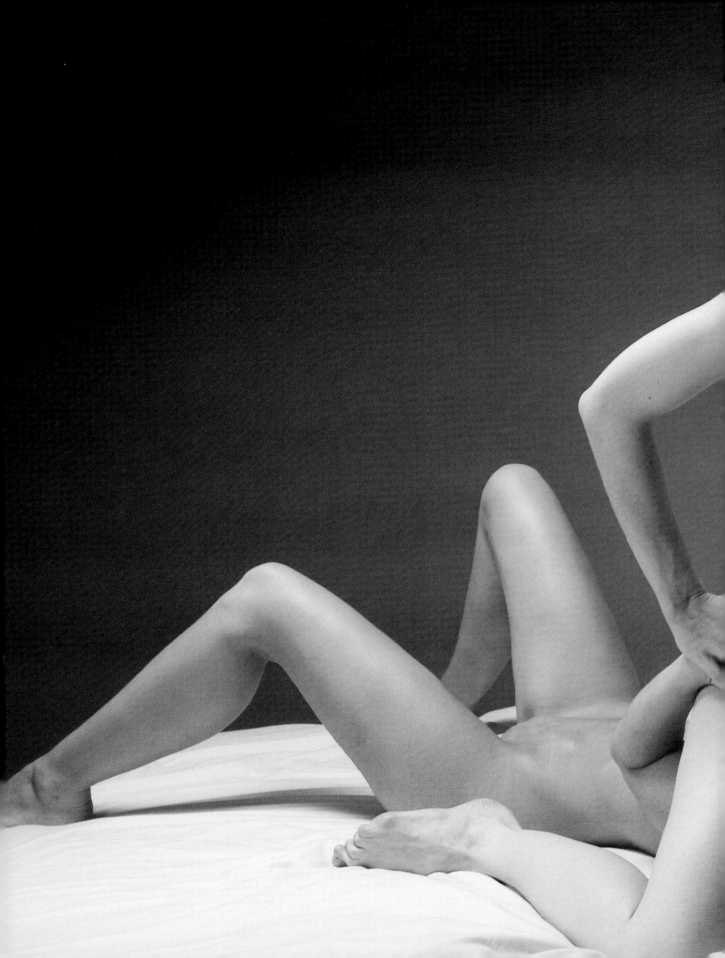

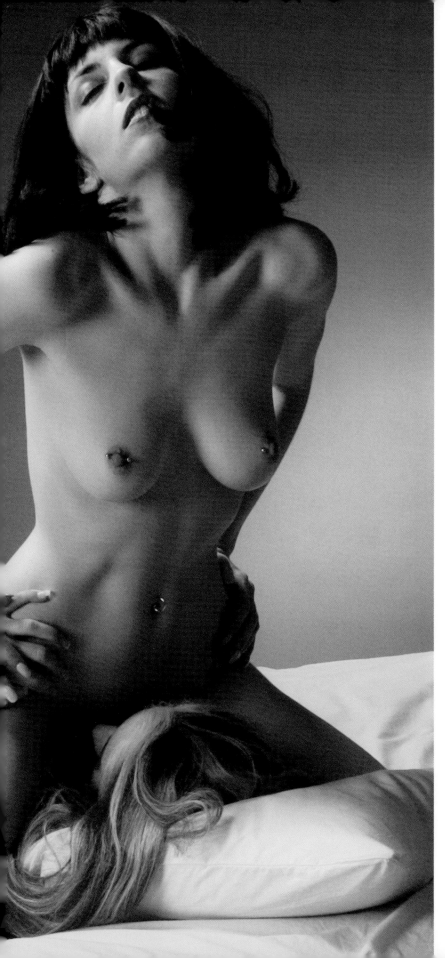

Taste receptor cells fire messages to our brain, the hub for all erotic activity. The brain interprets these sensory impulses and transmits messages about them to other parts of our body. Since the mouth contains thousands of taste buds capable of responding to every kiss and lick, our brains must get a real charge out of you tasting your lover and her tasting you.

Taste is actually a complex blending of the senses of taste and smell, meaning if you can't smell it, amazingly you won't be able to distinguish its taste. Therefore, her natural or enhanced scent will play a part in your overall kissing, licking, and tasting experience. Experiment with combinations of aromas as you orally enjoy one another. Simply lighting a scented candle or applying a new perfume behind your ears, in your cleavage, and on your thighs can elicit a newly succulent experience for both lovers.

Taste can be enhanced or suppressed. Suck. It will increase the flow of fluids. Saliva plays a huge role in gustatory adventures. It's not until whatever is in our mouth is wet with saliva can we begin to taste it. The saliva also spreads the flavors all over the tongue so your palate can discriminate with real gusto.

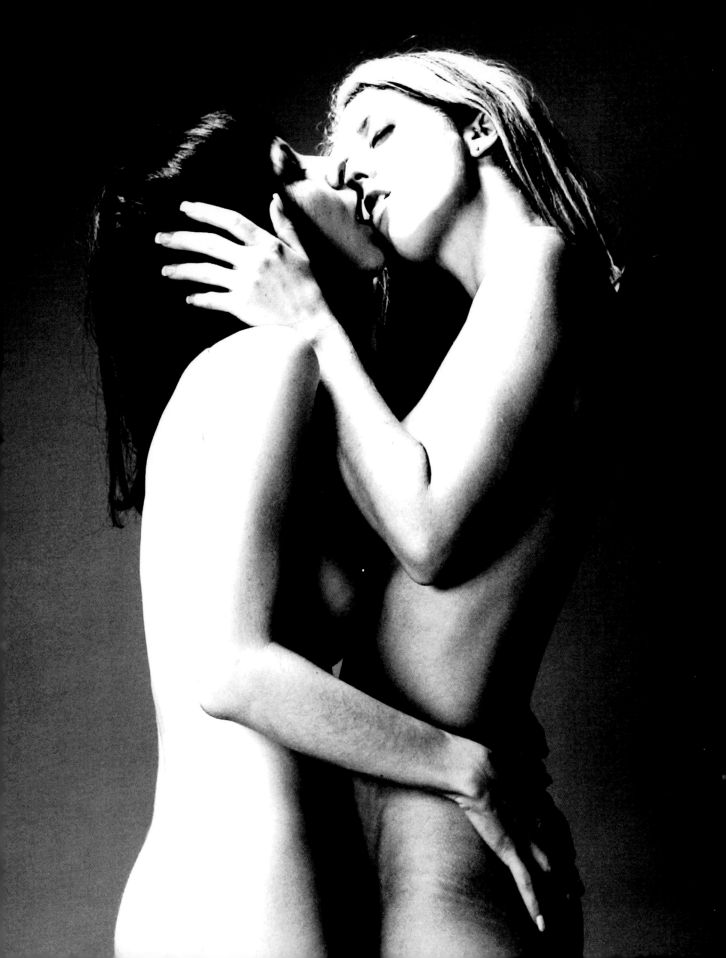

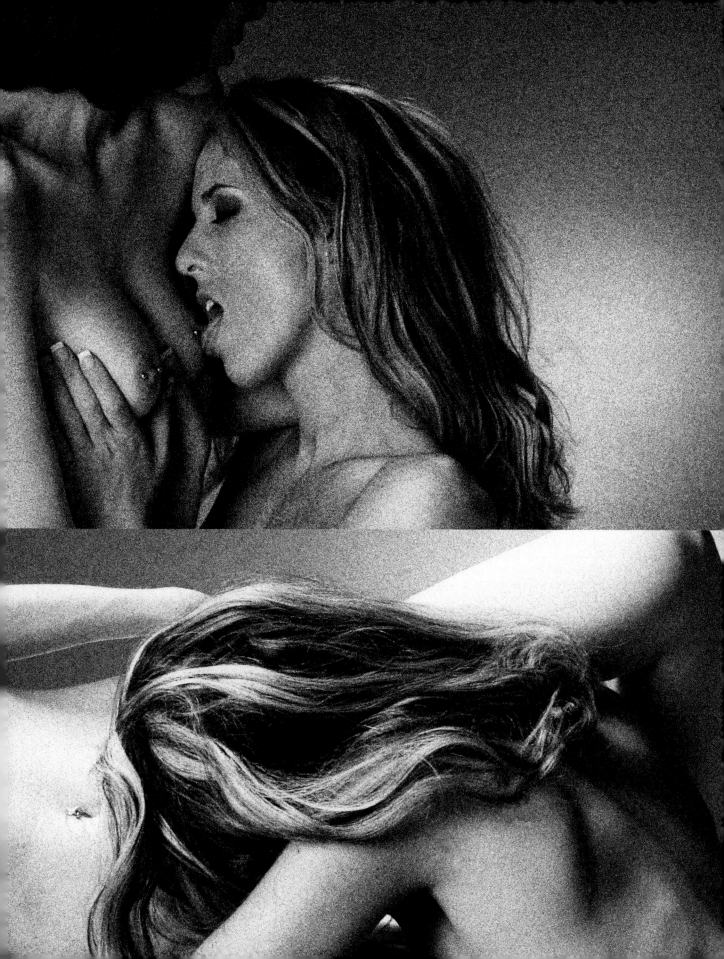

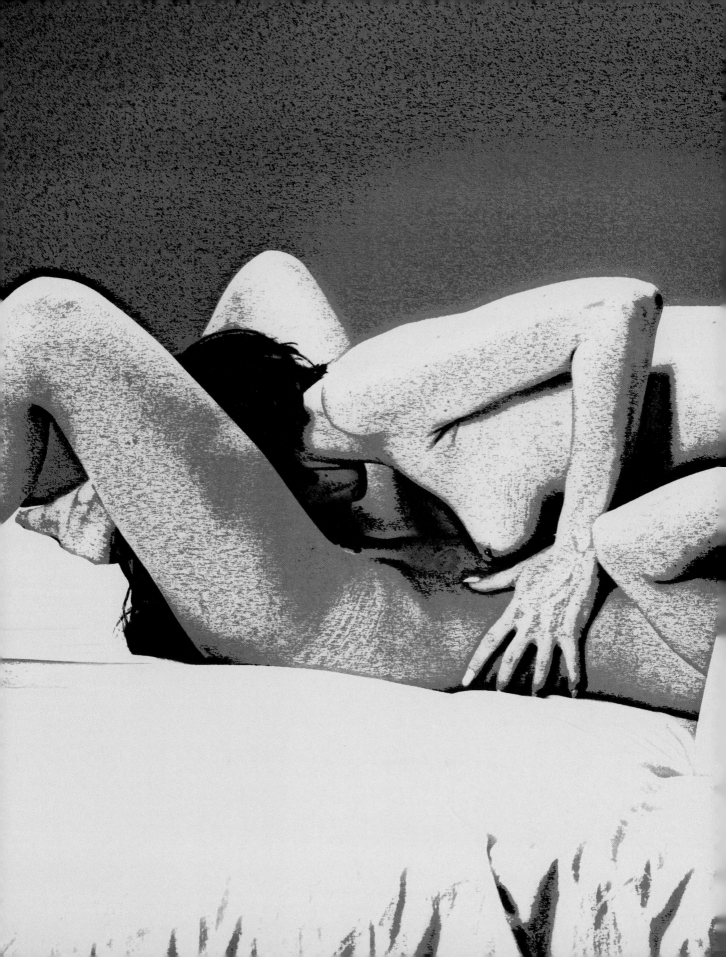

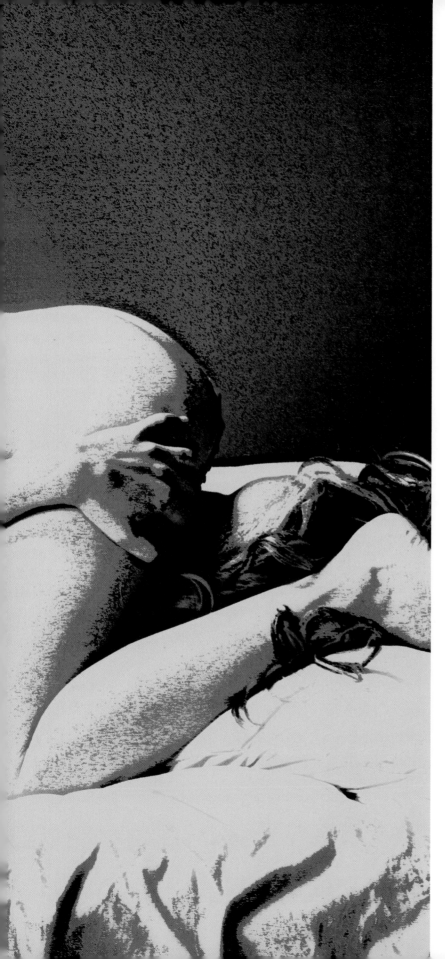

The same woman will taste different from one day to the next. During foreplay, lick and taste her everywhere — in and around the fingers, neck, eyelids, earlobe, her slit and her clit, under her arms, and in the nook of her elbow, to experience every taste du jour. Tasting one another is a major part of lovemaking, but if you're not into oral play as much as the next girl, apply a flavored lubricant first. Cleanliness and a healthy diet will help maintain a tasty pussy; avoid garlic, asparagus, alcohol, and strong, spicy foods before getting lucky.

When you go down on her after she has had a climax, you may notice that she tastes different now, perhaps saltier. We can taste salty, sour, sweet, bitter, or the less common umami, a more savory sensation involving certain proteins and amino acids. Our sense of taste protects us as spoiled foods taste sour and poison is usually bitter. Whether spoiled women taste sour or fatal women bitter is best left up to speculation!

The old school aphrodisiacs such as oysters and chocolate may not always impact sexual desire, but the simple act of feeding them to your lover is enough to boost the mood. And once we are granted permission to take a woman into our mouth to distinguish and revel in her flavor, we can truly lay claim to the unique sensory experience of tasting one of the finest delicacies the world's "ports of call" has to offer.

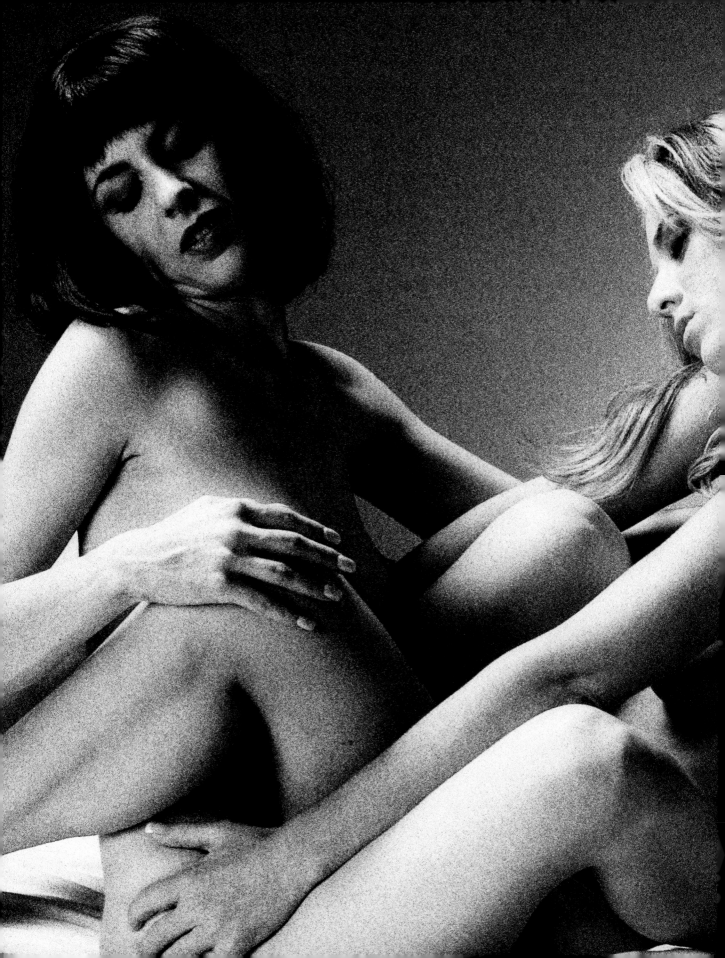

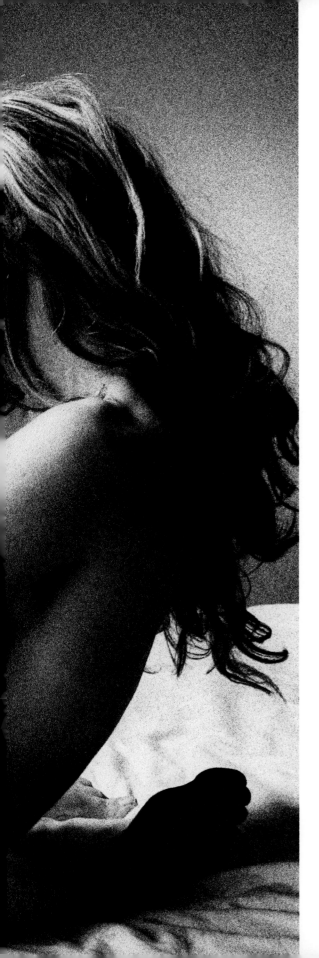

Pressure and friction create heat, and one of the best ways to generate sexual heat is to rub one's genitals. Tribade is an early term used to describe a woman rubbing on another woman to stimulate herself, mainly her clitoris and labia. Sappho wrote about women rubbing their clits, a pastime that continues as foreplay, and frequently leads to an orgasm.

rub

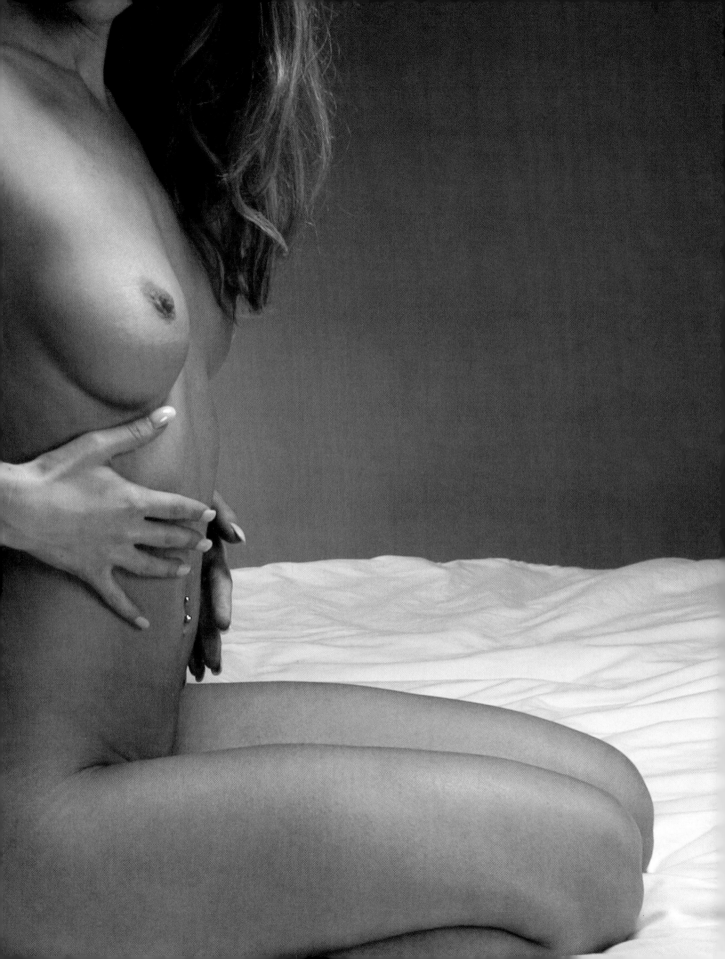

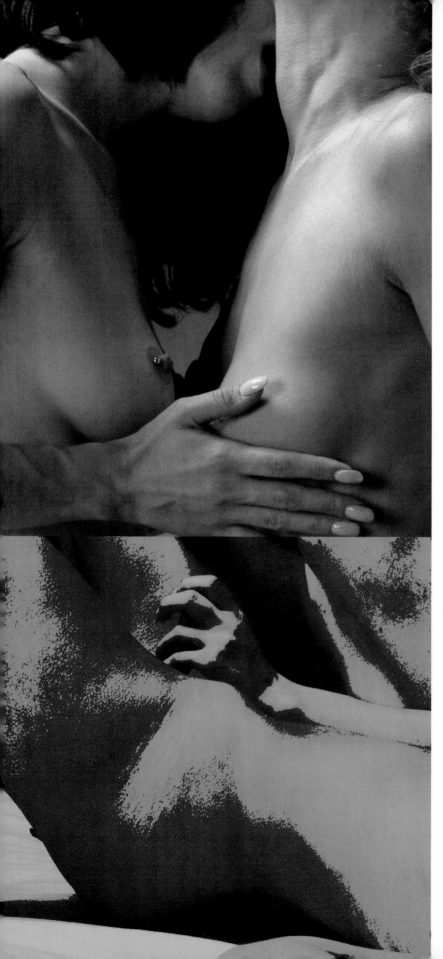

As children we find it completely natural to rub ourselves, and we come to realize that the rubbing feels good—that we have the capability to pleasure ourselves. Throughout our childhood we enjoy rocking horses, sliding down the banister, riding a bike, and climbing trees, perhaps straddling and lingering on a branch for a while. There's also the delight of discovering the jets of a swimming pool, sampling various stuffed animals, and the comfort of a favorite pillow.

Later in life, the jets and childhood toys take a back seat to the more convenient and efficient vibrator. In the late 1800s, vibrators were used as a medical device to soothe "hysteria" in women. But once the pornography industry took a liking to them in the early 1900s, polite women were unfortunately discouraged from partaking in the vibrator's obvious health benefits. In the last few decades, women have reclaimed the vibrator as a favorite accessory for autoeroticism.

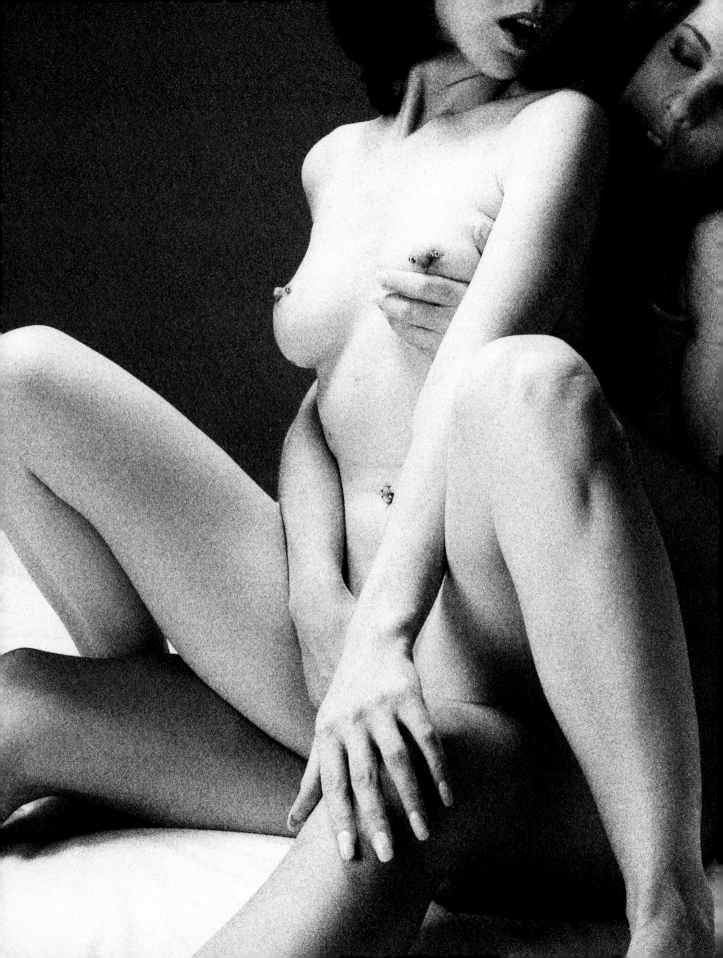

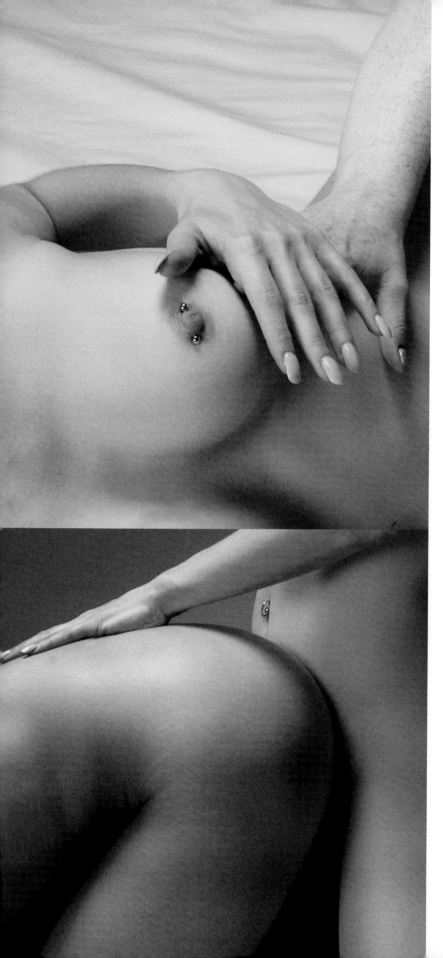

Women can become sexually aroused from the stroking of many areas of their bodies, including but not limited to the clitoral region, the breasts and nipples, and the feet. Each woman's clitoris varies in its rhythm and stroking preferences. Sometimes it will respond to fast and firm touch, other times the clitoris prefers to be caressed slowly and gently.

For heat and friction to grow into fire, oxygen is a vital component. In addition to finding yours and your lover's ultimate rhythm as you "buff the mrs." and grind your way to ecstasy, become aware of the rhythm of your breathing as you're making love. In particular, deep and steady breathing enables the mind and body to achieve the harmonic combination of arousal, tension, and relaxation necessary to reach a full body climax.

"Accidentally" brush against her when she least expects it. Or wake her up in the middle of the night by rubbing against her body. Never underestimate the thrill of surprise contact.

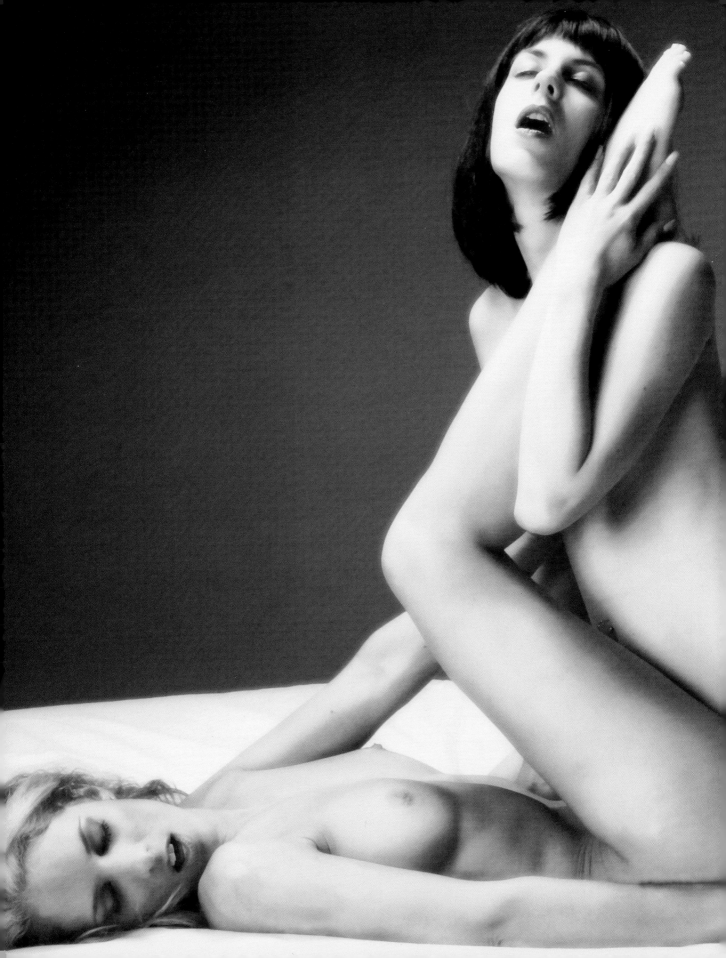

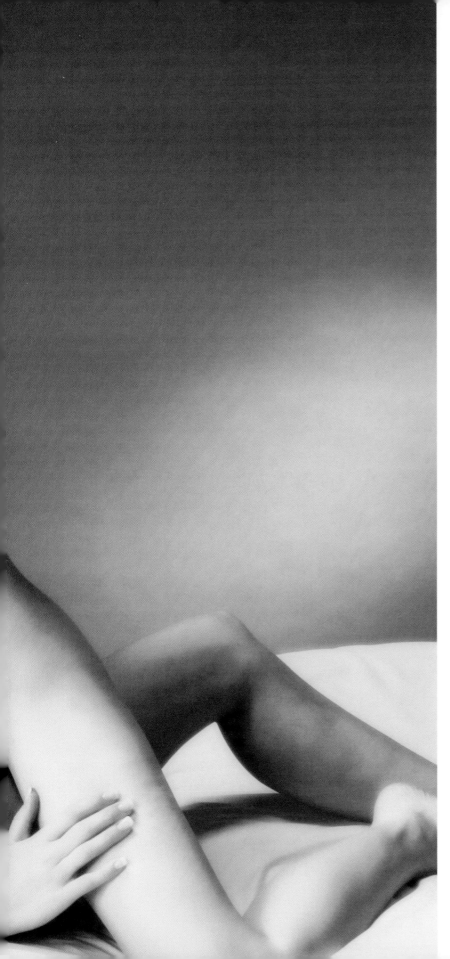

Rub on her thigh or foot while you pleasure her orally. As you give her a back massage, grind against her lovely ass. Let her flip you over onto your back and feel her wetness slowly rub up the length of your leg until her nipple tickles your clitoris. As afterplay, rubbing is a great way to indulge in an additional orgasm before the encounter winds down.

A truly intimate lovemaking act is to rub your clitoris against your lover's clitoris. This can be accomplished from many angles. One position for this full grind of clit against clit, pussy melting into hot pussy, has both women propped up on their hands or elbows, one lover twisting onto her side with her top leg draped over her lover's leg. The women spread and slide in until their pussies meet and rub, usually in a circular motion. This is a great way for lovers to attempt a simultaneous orgasm. As your hips swivel in unison, tell her as you draw close to your climax so she can pace and control her excitement and release herself with you.

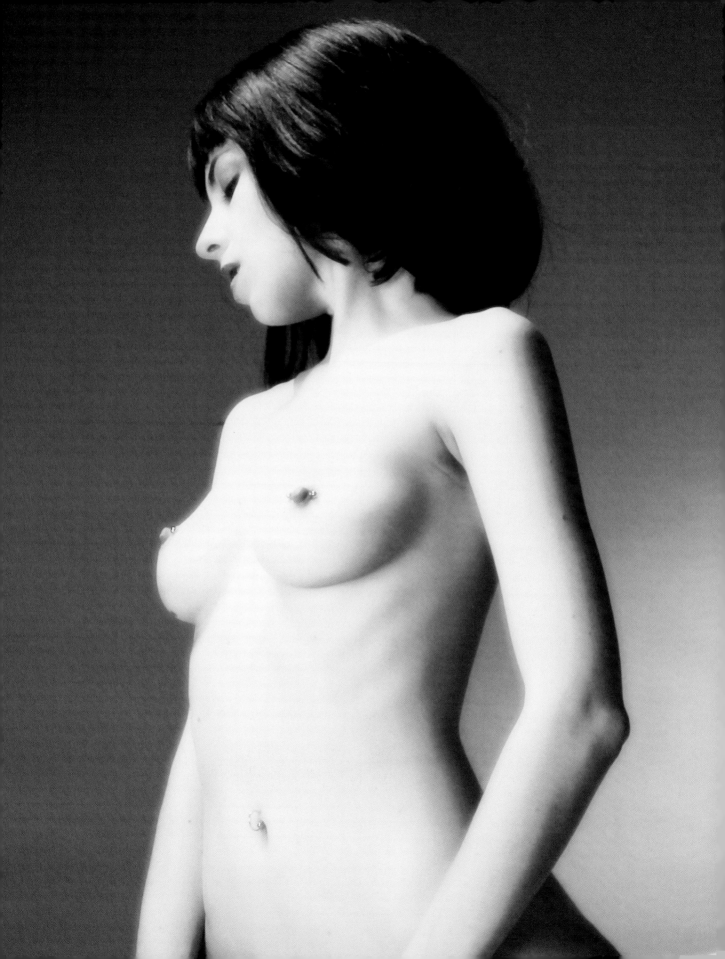

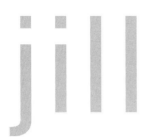

jill

Practice makes perfect, and to truly appreciate our capacity for pleasure, we must feel firsthand how our bodies respond to various stimuli. Pursuant to better understanding our own sensuality, we can learn to control our bodies and our lovemaking experiences so that our overall sexual enjoyment will intensify. The journey of self–awareness will begin when a woman literally takes herself into her own hands to masturbate, or what is more playfully referred to as "jilling off."

Women pride themselves on intuition, but thankfully no one can intuit your every desire, so first learn and enjoy yourself, then guide and share with a lover. A woman can stay in touch with herself as her body, sexual and emotional maturity, sex drive, and objects and pursuits of desire evolve over the years.

Self love is normal, natural, healthy, and fun. A culture of shame and embarrassment has created for some an enormous barrier to self–gratification. It's so natural to explore our bodies and stimulate our own genitals. Enjoy your body and strive to become the proud, sexual creature that recognizes and revels in the benefits of touching and pleasing herself. If you've been hesitating to enjoy the pleasures of masturbation, get a hold of yourself; your palms won't grow hair and you won't lose your ability to concentrate or reproduce. In addition to teaching us about sexual response and the feelings of pleasure it produces, masturbation promotes relaxation and relieves stress.

There's no one or right way to please ourselves. Women's bodies are all slightly different, and our moods fluctuate like the tides, so as with all sexual experiences, be flexible and willing to try different techniques, settings, and accessories. Fantasize or narcissize, whatever sparks your interest at that moment. Privacy affords privilege, and the ultimate privilege of masturbation is the ecstasy and release of a great orgasm.

Create an environment where you can focus on your body without distraction or discomfort. Become familiar with the shapes and textures of your obvious sexual hotspots; breasts and nipples, clitoris, vulva, labia, and vagina. Check yourself out in a mirror at different angles. Explore your not–so obvious hotspots like your neckline, sides and hips, buttocks and inner arm. As you discover yourself, apply lotions, oils, lubricant, or your own saliva to enhance the erotic stimulation. Toys, most typically vibrators, are a wonderful masturbation accessory. They offer the constant stimulation most women require to orgasm, and come in all shapes, textures, speeds, and sizes for convenience on the road or, home use.

Masturbation is not always a solo gig, and need not be confined to a dark bedroom. Mutual masturbation is when a woman stimulates both herself and her lover, or any combination thereof. It's part show with a dash of tell. If you've always wanted to watch your lover please herself, ask. Autoeroticize as you play voyeur. This ideal classroom setting allows you to learn about what she likes and how she likes it done. Or join in while she's visiting her mrs., adding extra fingers or your tongue to her usual self–love ritual.

Is masturbation sex? Let's put the matter to bed; of course masturbation is sex.

After a long day I love to come home, soak in a hot bath and jill off with my hand shower. The tried–and–true 'waterworks' is my favorite tension reliever. I'm relaxed, fresh and ready to climb into bed.

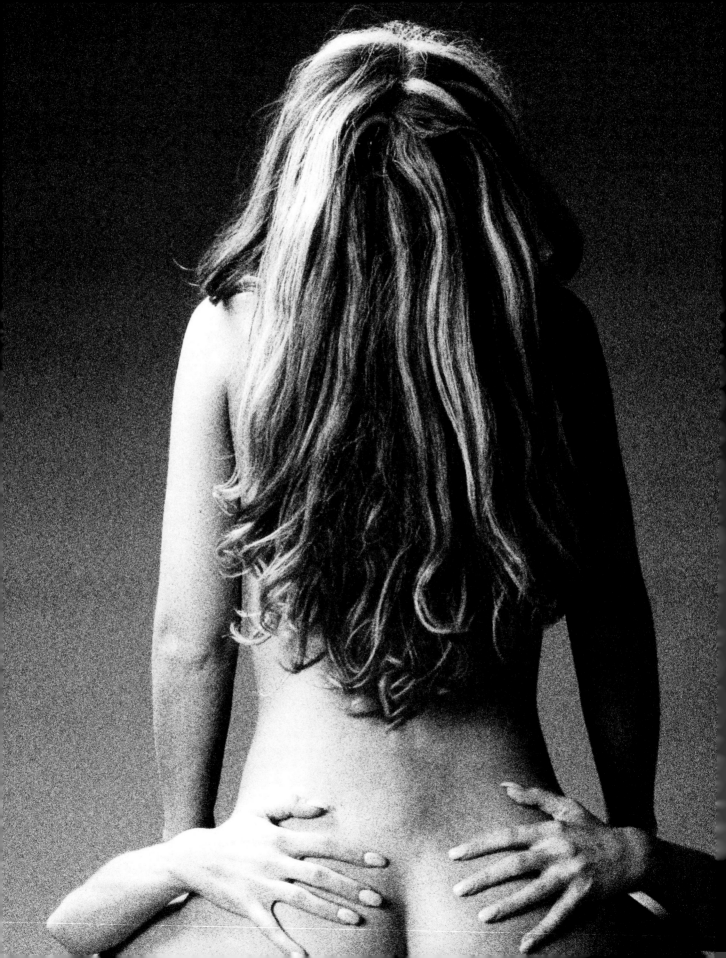

We are inquisitive creatures with a natural passion to experience what seems exotic to us. With regard to sex, striving to experience the new can be intimidating. Step one is the willingness to toss our fears to the wayside, break out of our sexual comfort zone, and try. Be adventurous and bold. Give it a whirl. Actively pursue the delightful possibilities that lie within your untapped erotic imagination.

spice

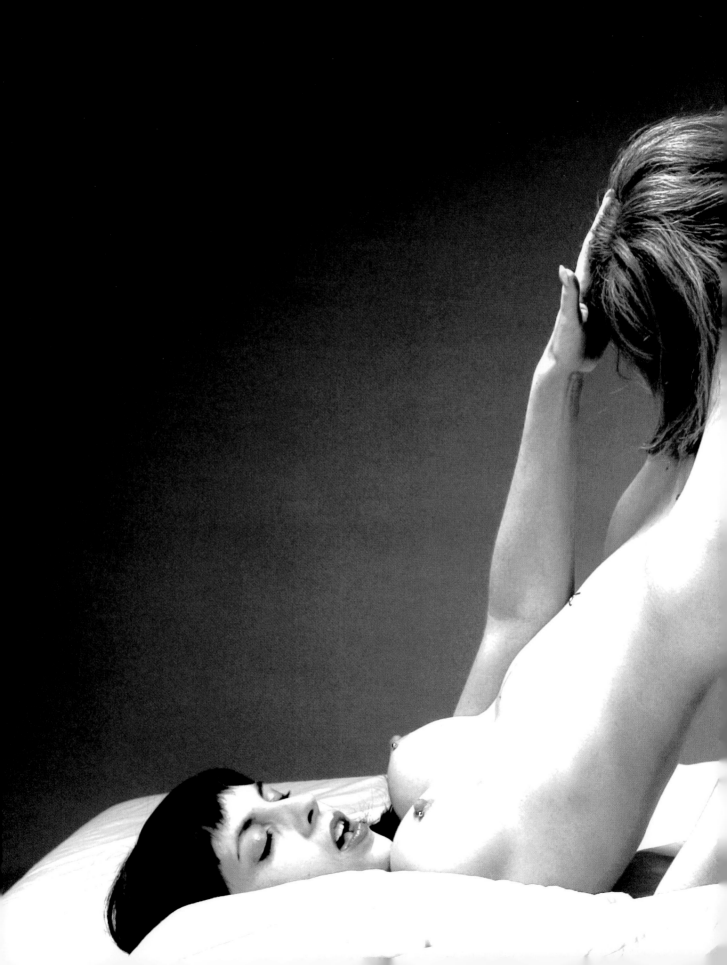

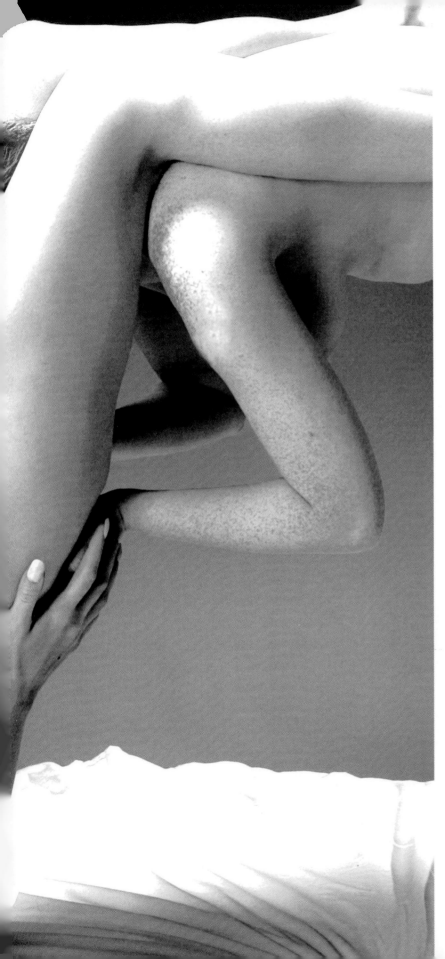

What arouses your interest? To spice up your sex life you must first acknowledge your curiosities. Test the waters. Sometimes revitalizing the passion is as simple as going down on her from a new, different angle. Look at racy photos. How do they make you feel? Share them with your lover to instigate dialogue and determine her receptiveness for trying something new. Imagery stimulates the often overlooked but extremely potent and demanding sex organ, the mind.

Teasing is a light spice. Playfully undress for your lover. Anxiousness can cause you to rush the show. Let her have a peek but don't reveal all the goods at once or too quickly. Anticipation is electrifying.

The unexpected provides a rush synonymous with sexual arousal. Trim your bush into a heart-shape, a star, an inviting landing strip, or allow her initials to mark the spot, perhaps even going completely bare on your lower lips. Without a word, take her hand and place it on your newly shorn pussy. Shaving and being shaved can also be a spicy variety of foreplay.

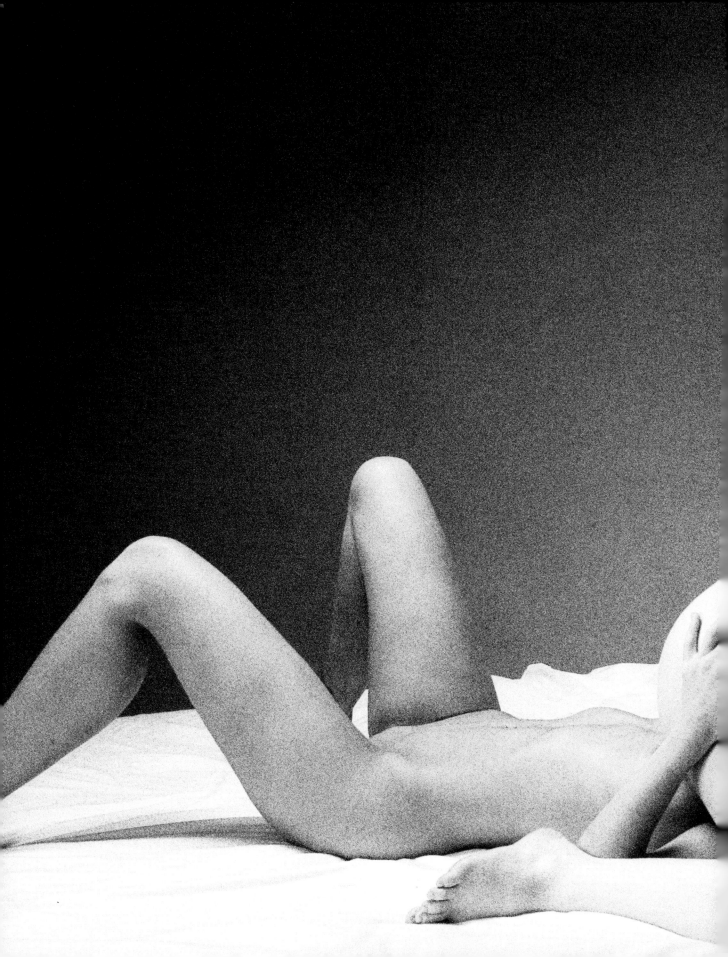

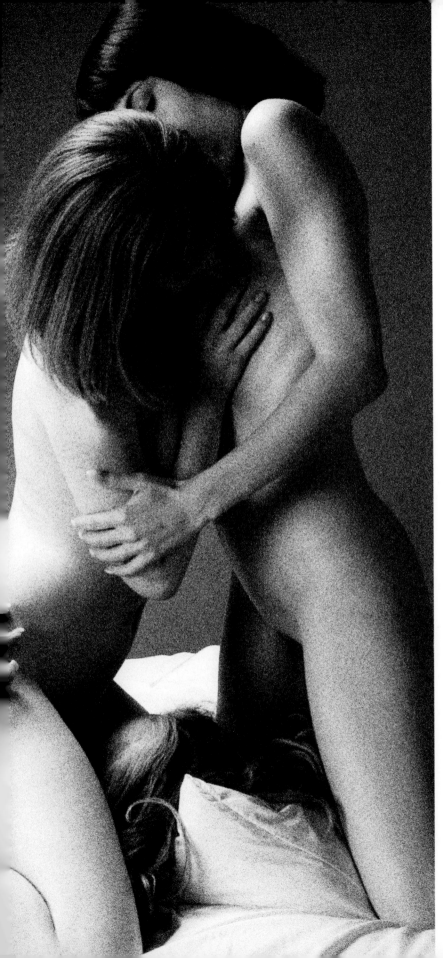

The best fantasy has a hint of possibility. This is true even if your fantasy is to do something you would never act out in reality. Beyond the sexual turn-on benefits of fantasizing are the additional and often surprising intellectual, emotional, and spiritual responses you can have as you discover and ponder a previously hidden or undeveloped side of yourself. You can spice up your sex life by both sharing your fantasy with your lover or keeping it all to yourself. The simple act of freeing your mind and allowing yourself to imagine yourself doing what you consider to be excitingly unusual or different stimulates your potential to enjoy sex more fully.

Have you fantasized about being with two girls at once? Meet a new friend and invite her over for a ménage á trois. The thrill of twenty fingers, two tongues, and a trio of pussies is unparalleled.

Role playing releases us of our inhibitions and nurtures deeper feelings of trust and intimacy between lovers. It can be spontaneous or scripted. Try goddess and slave, victim and rescuing heroine, or saucy tramp and virtuous virgin. There's also nature girl and urban temptress, MaryAnn and Ginger, or the ever-popular Mistress and her French maid.

Never underestimate the power of romance and attentiveness when the flames of desire need fanning. Romance is linked with the hormones oxytocin and vasopressin, which produce the happy feelings we get from the natural stimulants dopamine and serotonin. Light her fire with flowers, a card with a handwritten poem, candles, and other delicate touches to show your partner that she is special. Treat her to a luxurious sponge bath.

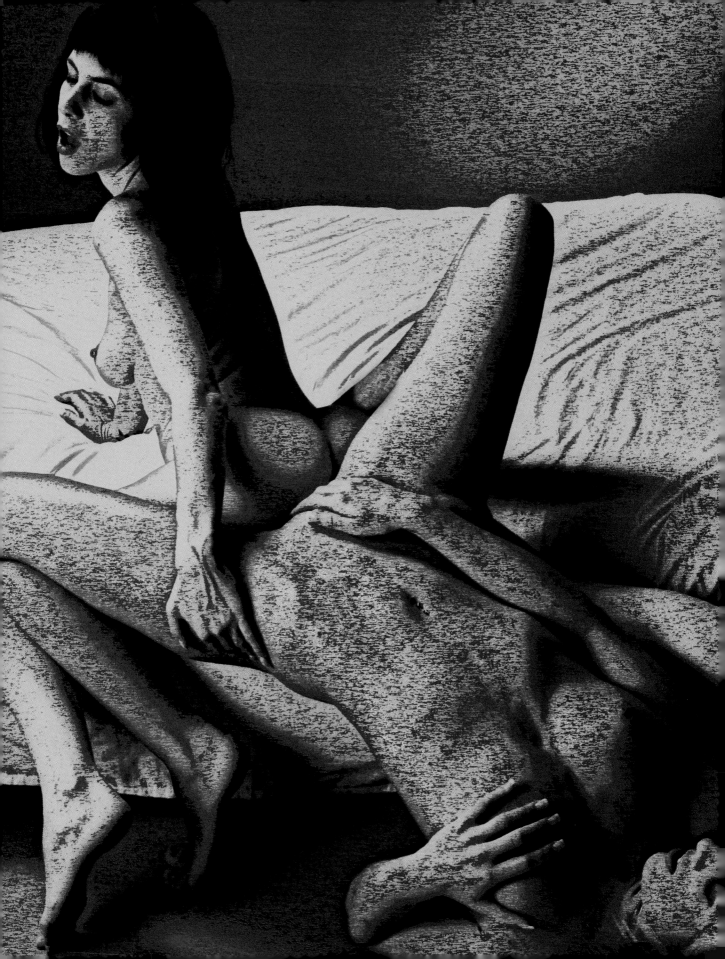

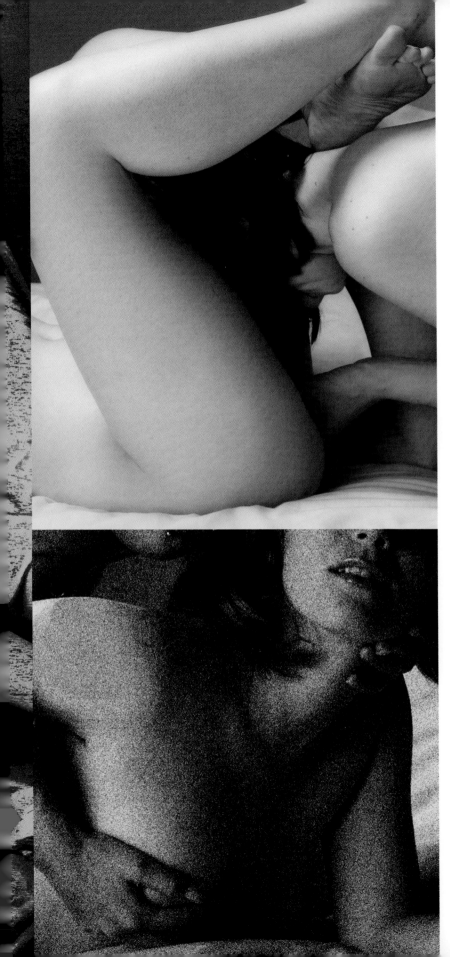

Are you usually timid and quiet during sex? Tonight, yell out loud. Been wearing those same old baggie jammies, frumpy robe, fluffy slippers or sweat pants? Don a tool belt and see if it floats her boat. Surprise her by wearing a sexy nighty. Make yourself irresistible. Spritz her with an extravagant perfume. Make an occasion out of no occasion at all. Add a sexy pair of heels to make your legs look especially shapely. Heels also provide the added, stimulating ingredient of authority.

Is she usually the "top?" Tonight utterly dominate her. Tops, bottoms, and switching are not about ego, but about trust and empowerment resulting from the roles of dominating or submitting, wholly. Take charge and ravish her or for once, allow yourself to totally succumb. The feeling can be new and marvelous.

Getting sexy on atypical surfaces can spice up the loving. Go down on her as she sits on the washer and spreads her legs for the duration of the spin cycle. Pass her a note telling her to meet you in the back seat of your sedan in five minutes. Pop in your favorite driving music and enjoy the ride.

Props—even a simple wig, jewelry, or henna tattoos—add to the fun, so take the time to accessorize. Atmosphere is also important. Even though you and your lover are the sole audience, by setting the stage for your performances you reinforce how important it is to please one another. Above all, don't take it all too seriously. Achieving and maintaining a constantly innovative and dynamic love life is tricky business. What's most important is to enjoy the journey.

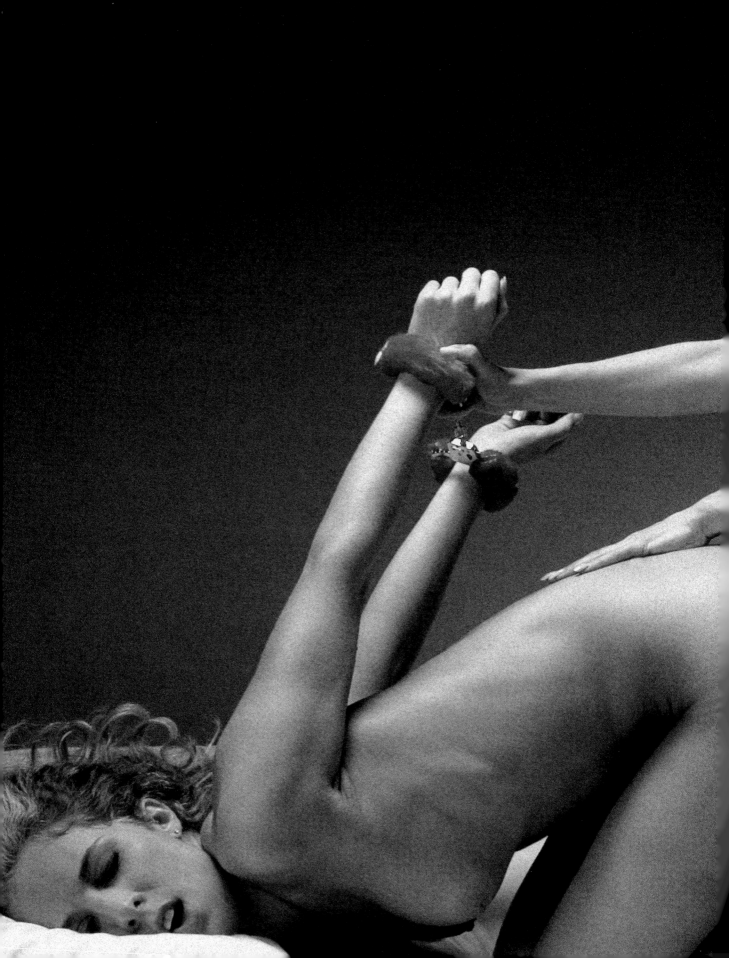

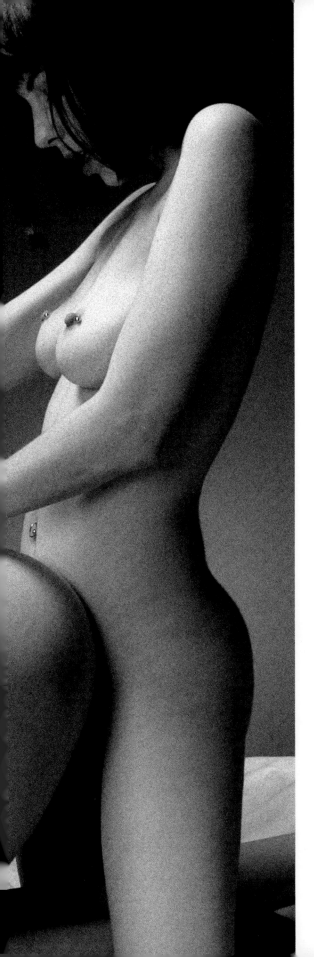

Kinkiness describes particular sexual urges and behaviors that appeal to more unconventional tastes. The lure in performing sexual activities that involve fetish, bondage, discipline, dominance, submission, and sadomasochistic activities is unique for everyone. Facing the forbidden is thrilling and acting out what intrigues and intimidates us can make us stronger and more free both from sexual inhibitions and in other aspects of our lives where we are overly reticent.

kink

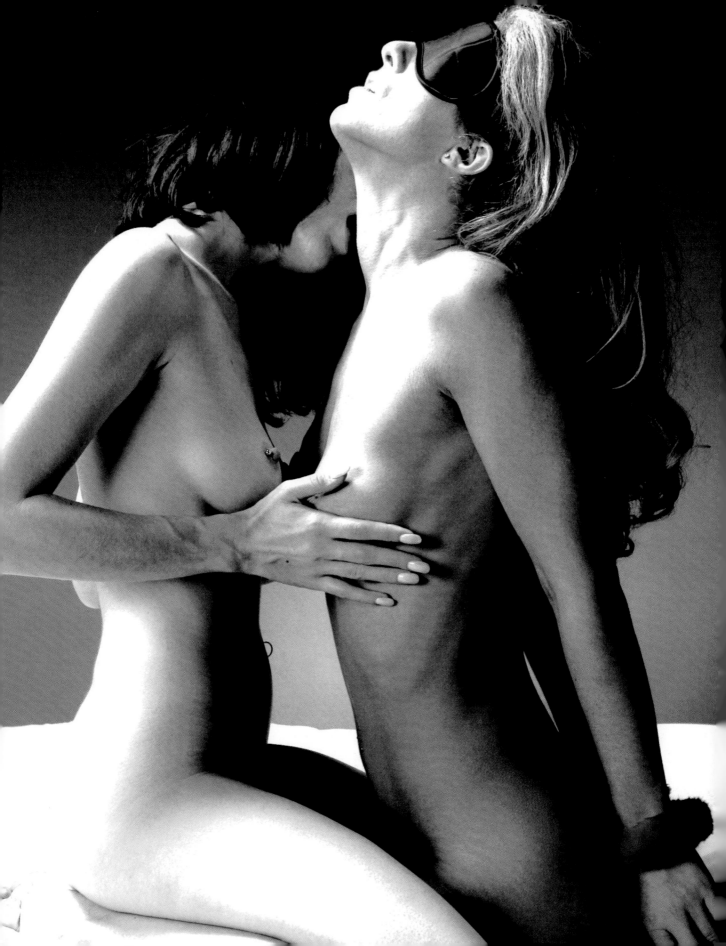

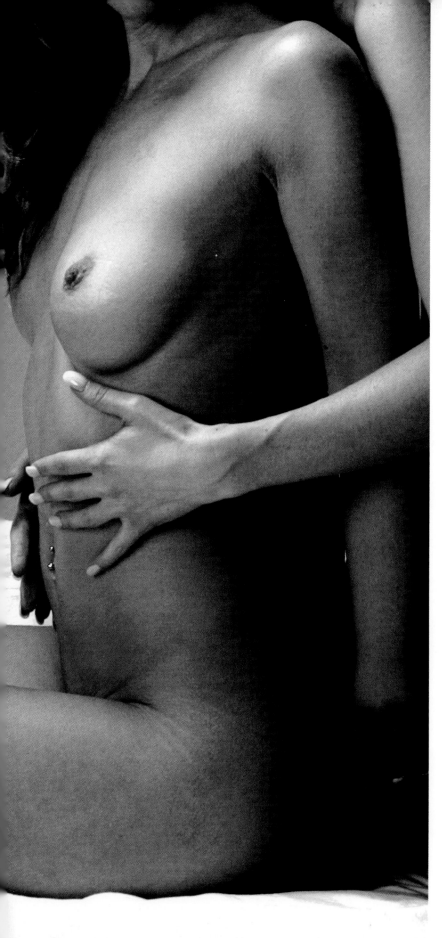

To discover what particular kink is for you will require confidence. Initially one may experience more variation with multiple lovers, but exclusive couples have the advantage of familiarity with their lover's body and its responses, and will better know their lover's preferences, all of which results in more consistently satisfying sex. As women grow comfortable with their sexuality and become more open-minded, adventurous, and courageous, and willing to overcome what they previously considered to be taboo, they can better realize and ultimately manifest what truly turns them on and subsequently will lead to the most gratifying sex.

Fetish often answers to aesthetics. If you have a fetish for cybersex, kitchen utensils, sploshing in the backseat of a muscle car, or erotic footplay involving stilettos, you owe it to yourself to explore these inclinations as the deepest sexual and personal fulfillments may result from allowing yourself to enjoy this taboo bliss. Perhaps piercings are your fixation. Tug, suckle, tweak, and attach yourself to the rings in her tongue, nipples, belly button, and genitals, or bars in the folds of her vulva. Piercings enhance sexual stimulation and make a pronounced fashion statement.

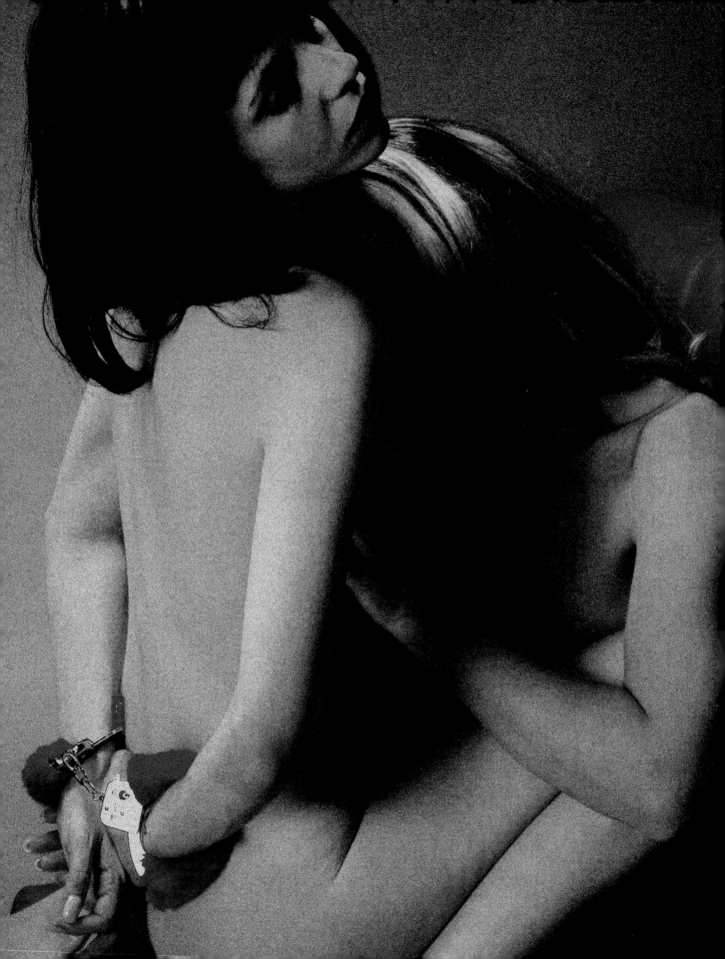

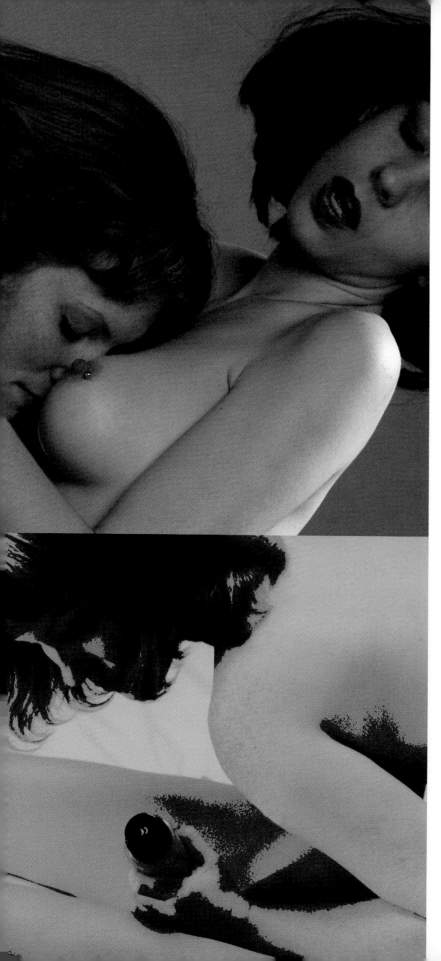

Power has been declared the ultimate aphrodisiac. This may link more directly to prosperity, which is sexy, but it also equates to dominance. Much of BDSM (Bondage, Domination, Submission, and Masochism) activity is related to power exchange. Many dominants enjoy the conspicuous, ostentatious behavior afforded in this showy role. Submissives may gain some relief from their everyday responsibilities, or perhaps get off on testing and impressing the dominant with their endurance. They also bask in the attention afforded to the role, and the thrill could be as simple as fulfilling a deep desire to serve. Cup your hand for the best sound as you teach your saucy girl a lesson with a firm spanking on her bare bottom. A hairbrush or wooden spoon will also relay your message. Traditional costumes such as leather corsets, masks, and thigh–high latex boots add to the atmosphere and facilitate our ability to fall into the role.

For most people, sexuality and gender identity lie on a bell curve rather than neatly at one or the other end of a spectrum. Cross–dress and gender–bend to explore the duality of both your feminine and masculine sides. Girl–on–girl blow jobs are pretty kinky, and sucking her strap–on cock is as much fun to watch as it is to do. It depends on the aggressiveness of the blower, but in general the receiver is more apt to climax if she simultaneously uses a vibrator on her clitoris for constant stimulation while being blown. Strap on a dildo to extend your clit for a girlie titty fuck. Similar to a blow job, this wild love act enables the recipient's clitoris the special experience of begin coddled and pumped within her lover's glistening cleavage.

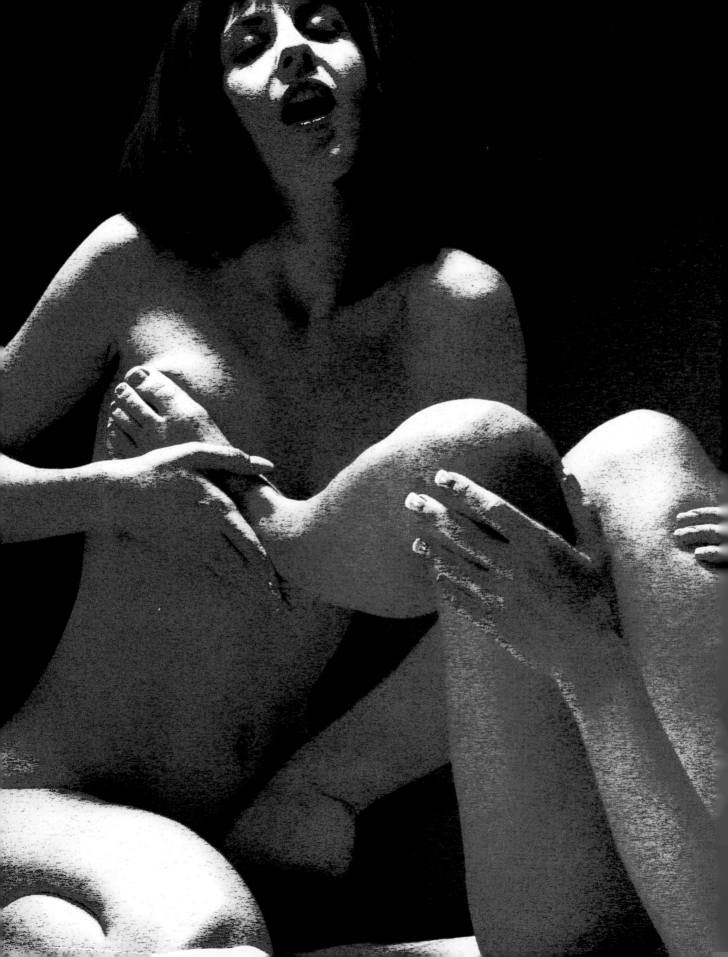

Sexuality is a powerful force in human consciousness and must be respected as such. Both pain and pleasure may release feel-good endorphins. Inflicting small doses of pain does not mean inflicting injury, and this level of kink is not for everyone. Be safe, sane, consensual, and respect the trust that's been established and the boundaries agreed–upon and safe words that have been negotiated and agreed upon. Seek professional advice regarding props and techniques when applicable. As you continue to celebrate your developing sexuality, proudly wear the label of kinky because you found a new way to do it today.

.

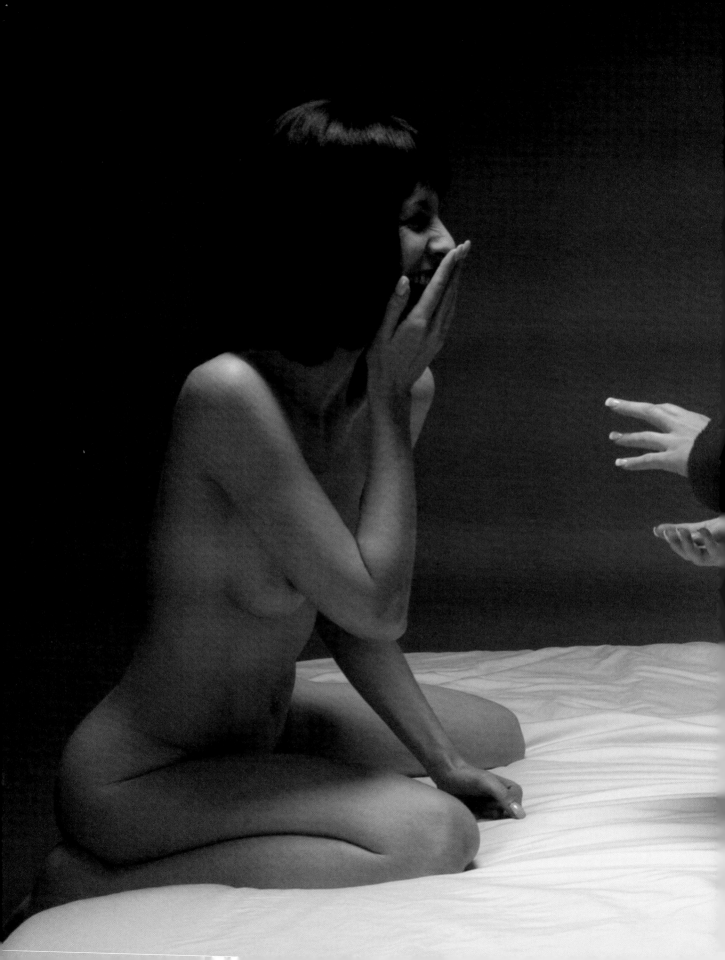

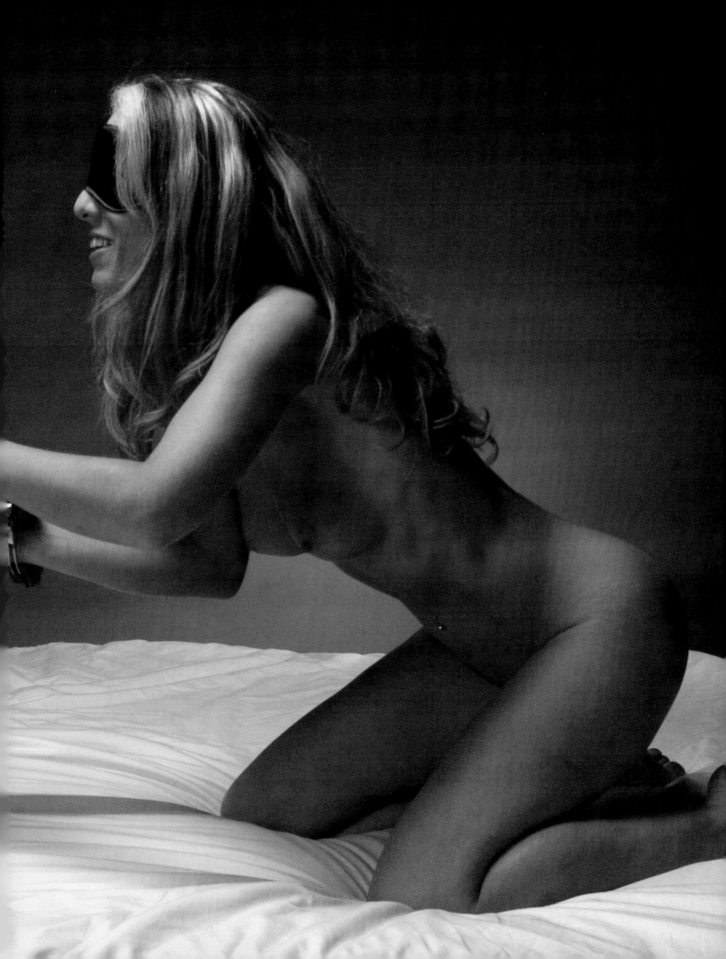

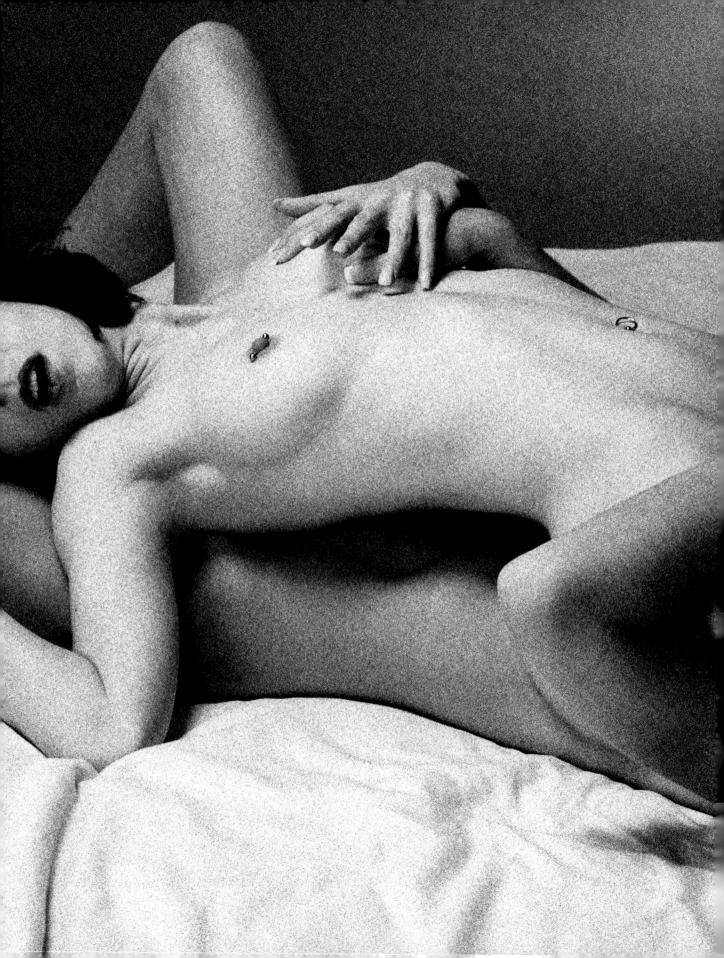

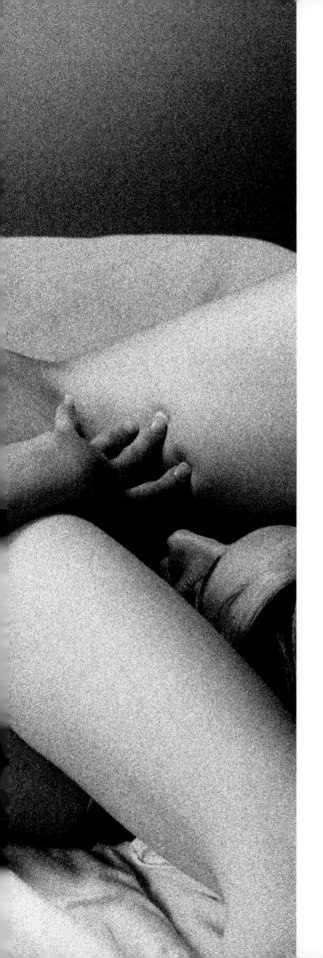

The power of the pussy can be daunting. It invites and incites all sorts of behavior, anxieties, fantasies, and myths. The history of the word "pussy" is vague, but for at least 100 years it has been applied, notably as a double entendre in the entertainment world, to anything soft and furry, tamed or untamed, whether this be a cat, a vulva, or a plant, the pussy willow leaping to mind.

pussy

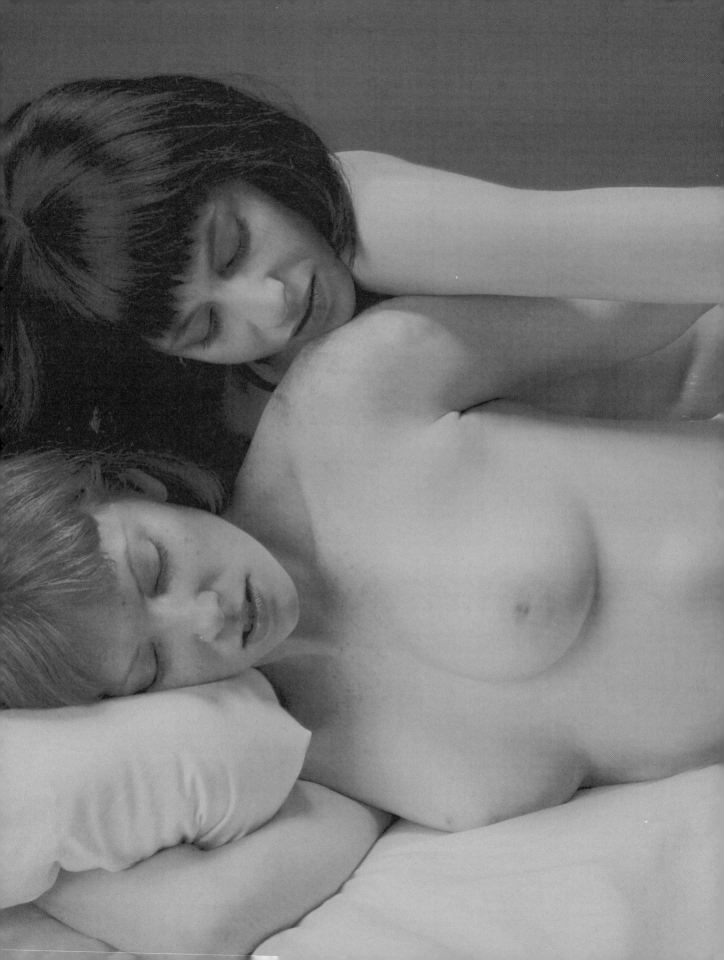

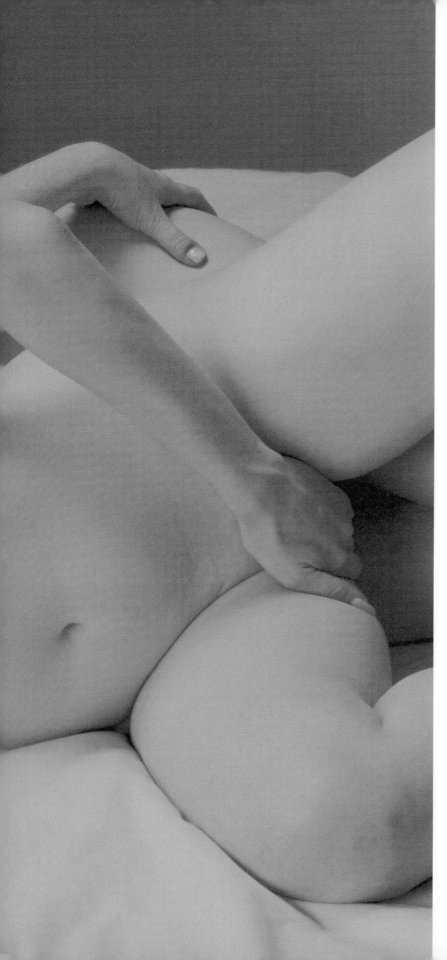

The basics of the pussy begin with the vulva, which refers to a woman's collective external genitalia. On either side of the vaginal vestibule are two sets of lips, the labia minora and the labia majora. The minora are two soft folds of skin within the majora. Vagina, the Latin word for "sheath" as in a tight-fitting protective covering, is the internal structure or pathway that connects the vulva to the cervix and uterus. This muscular tube usually runs about 4 inches, of which the first one-third is the most sensitive to erotic stimulation.

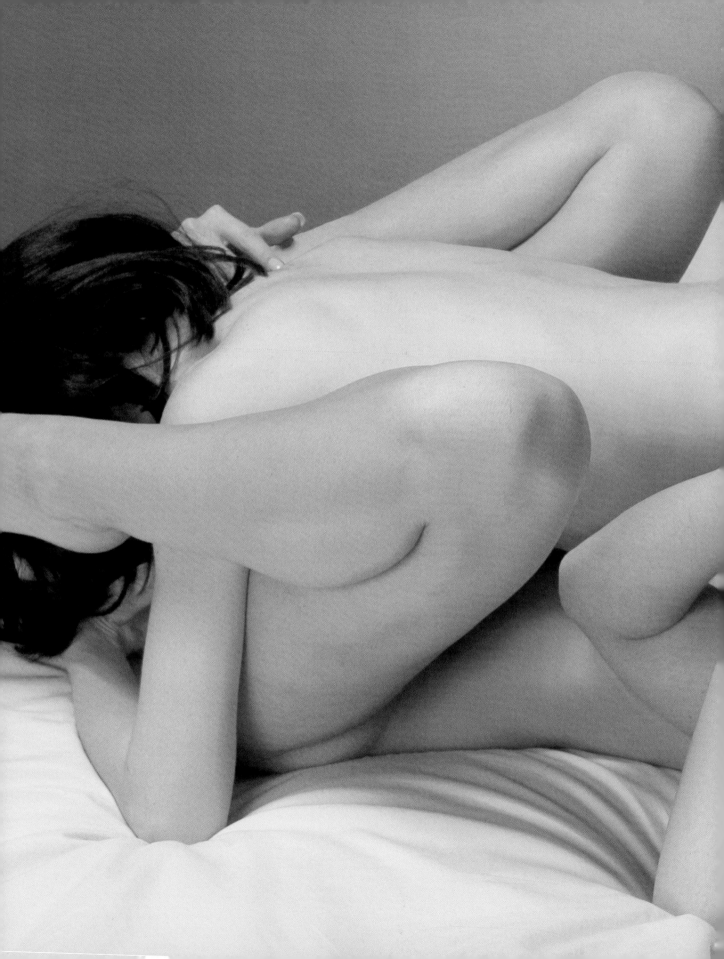

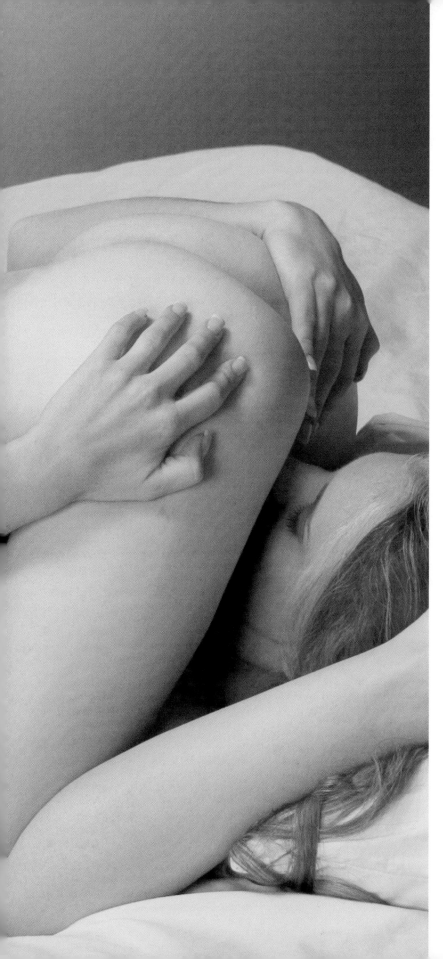

Within and along the front of the vaginal canal lies a woman's potentially ultra-sensitive urethral or perineal sponge, commonly known as her "g-spot." This mass of erectile tissue (it's not really a spot at all) can produce intense climaxes for some women when properly stimulated. The g-spot is named for Ernest Gräfenberg, a German doctor who wrote about this region in 1950, although he was far from the first to do so. Acknowledgement of the g-spot's existence can be traced back to early Chinese texts among other writings.

The pussy holds our most sensitive sex organ, the clitoris, the external portion of which is located above the vaginal canal at the front of the vulva where the labia minora meet. Thanks to the sexual revolution, in the last few decades the clitoris has overcome the blatant repressive tactics of those who have concealed the truth about the clit for so long.

For years medical texts more or less described the clitoris as a miniscule bump, the function and internal portions of which were rarely or barely acknowledged at all. In actuality, the clitoris is an erectile organ very homologous to the penis except that the sole function of the clitoris seems to be to provide sexual pleasure and release. The clitoris can be stimulated many ways and with varying degrees of firmness to suit a woman's unique desire.

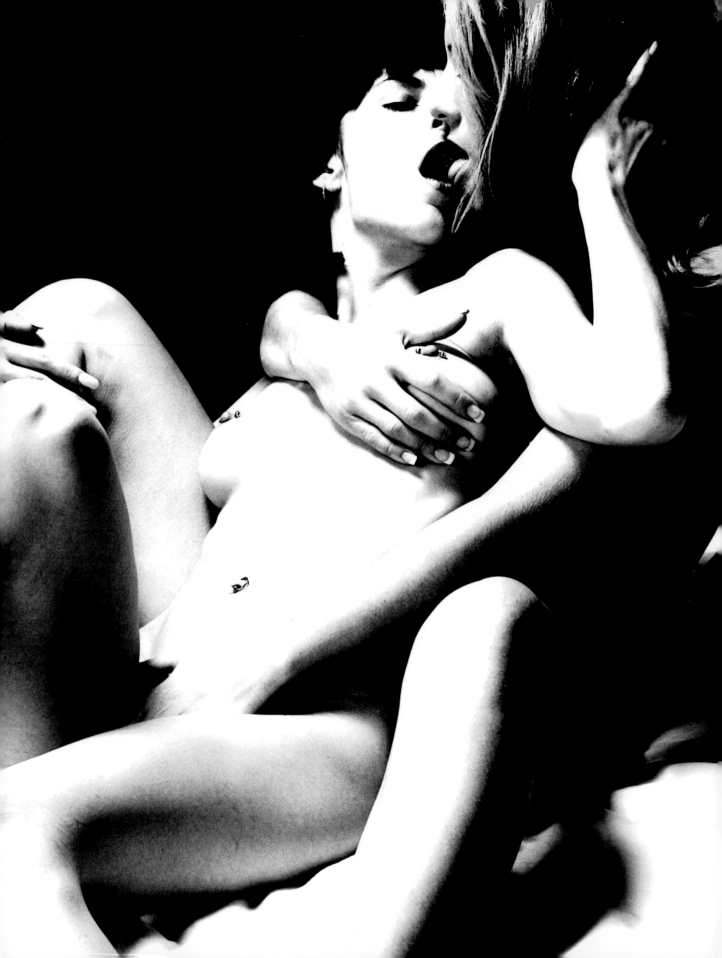

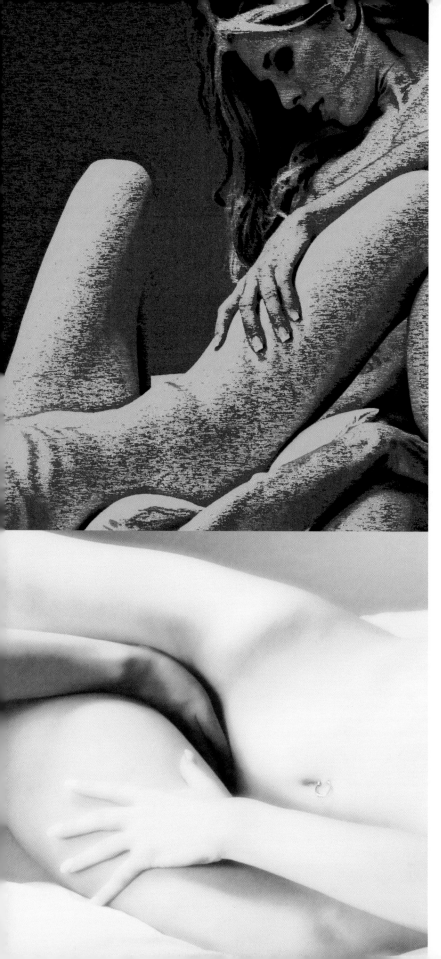

The pussy wants and needs to be exercised. Sexual stimulation tightens and tones the vagina, and lubrication keeps the vulva and vagina healthy and soft. You also get a vaginal workout when you start and stop your urination flow by contracting or squeezing and then relaxing primarily your pubococcygeus (PC) muscle. Repeat this throughout the day at varying intervals and speeds, sometimes clenching and releasing quickly, sometime squeezing and holding for a few seconds before the release. In addition to preventing incontinence and keeping the vagina taut and strong, this workout can improve the duration and intensity of your climaxes.

Every pussy has a unique personality and will behave and respond differently, often unexpectedly, in various contexts. We will discover with sexual experience that the pussy can be very fussy and at other times rather easy to please. Most women enjoy a steady and circular motion of rubbing on their clitoris. You can also flit your tongue on the clitoris and explore the entire pussy region with your mouth and tongue.

Place your mouth on her pussy and hum. This natural vibrator allows the tongue a brief break without cooling off the lovemaking. Just as your lover begins to climax, press on the clitoris with your fingers or tongue and hold there throughout the orgasm. This is an exceptional way for you to share in the waves of pleasure that she is feeling.

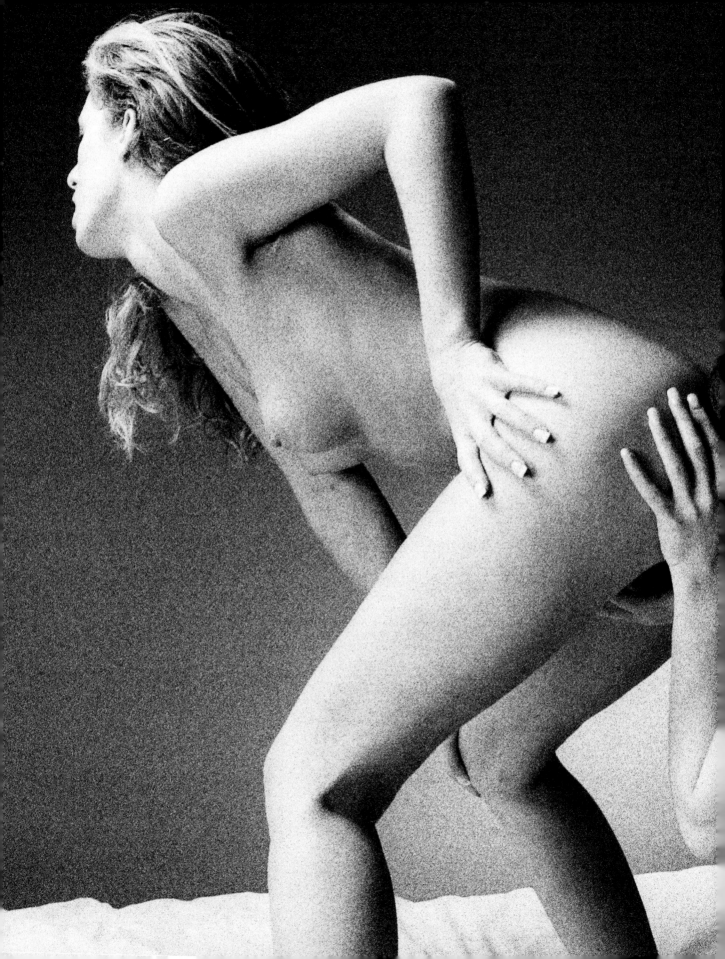

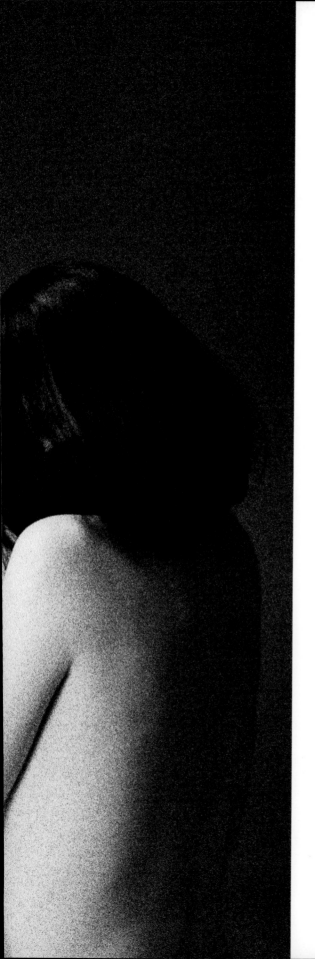

A lot of stock is put into the value of a nice ass, yet that same ass is all too frequently overlooked when prioritizing erogenous zones. Butts can be licked and kissed, massaged, stroked, lightly bitten, squeezed, spanked, and penetrated. The consensus of those who regularly engage in anal sex is that the sexual rewards are richer and the experience more intimate than imaginable.

ass

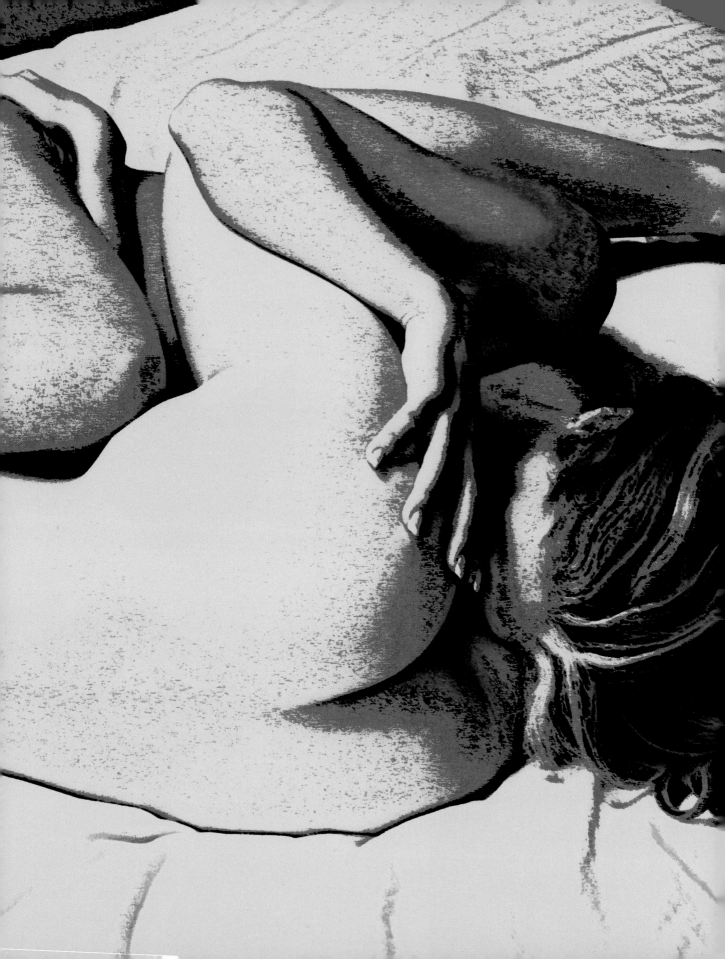

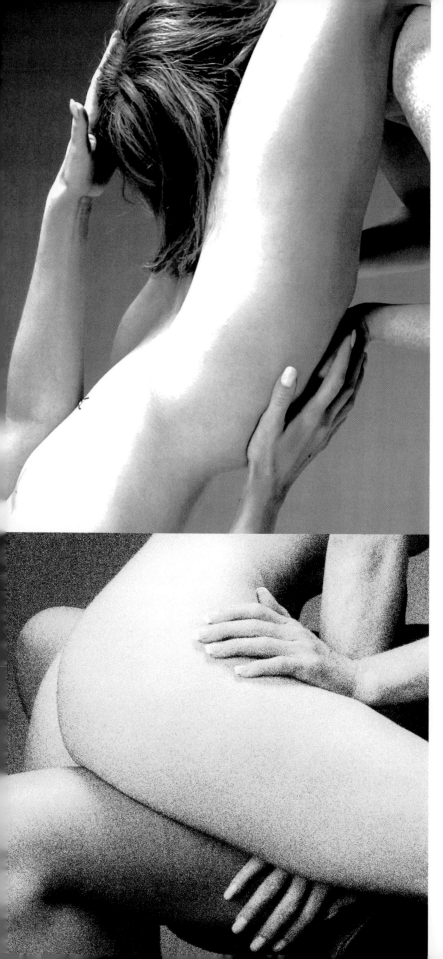

Newcomers can get friendly with their neglected and misunderstood asshole by fingering it in the shower. Explore and test responses of different regions in and around the anus. The depth of penetration is not the key here. Like the clitoris and labia, blood rushes to the many nerve endings in this region when aroused, and an aroused anal region eagerly enlarges in anticipation of further attention.

The basics of anal sex are lubrication, hygiene, relaxation, and pacing. Regardless of the arousal level, the ass is not self-lubricating, so buy the right lube and use plenty of it. Whether using fingers, the tongue, a dildo, butt plug, or anal beads, penetrate slowly as the pace of dilation allows. Communicate with your partner throughout, and if nervousness or discomfort overshadows the pleasure, or if it hurts, stop. Vary the position if the first one you try isn't comfortable. From behind may be best for one woman while another might prefer to be on her back or side.

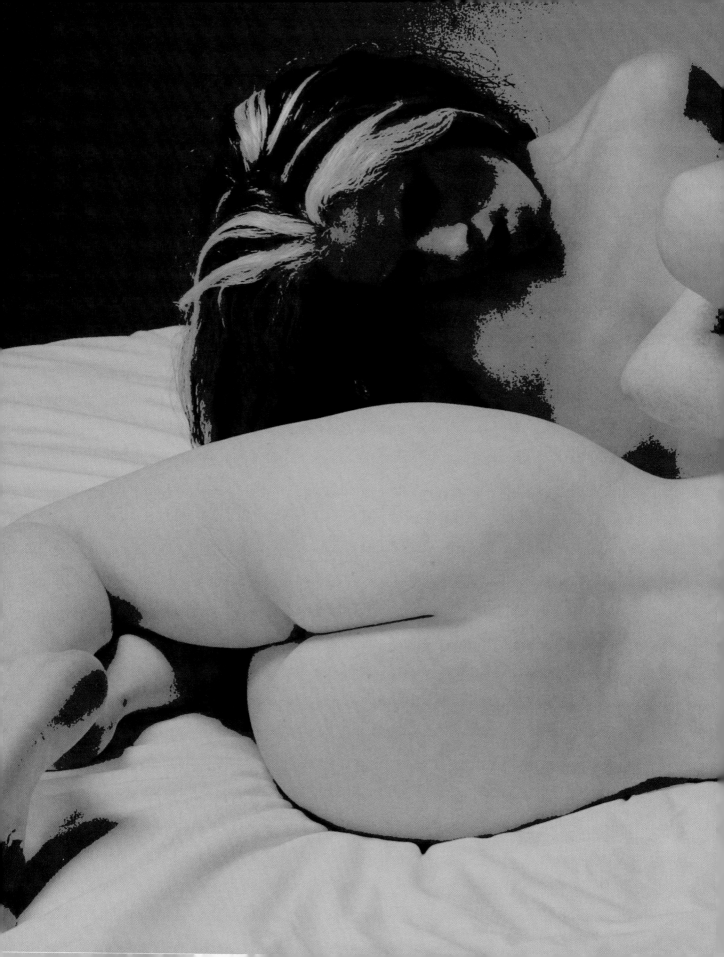

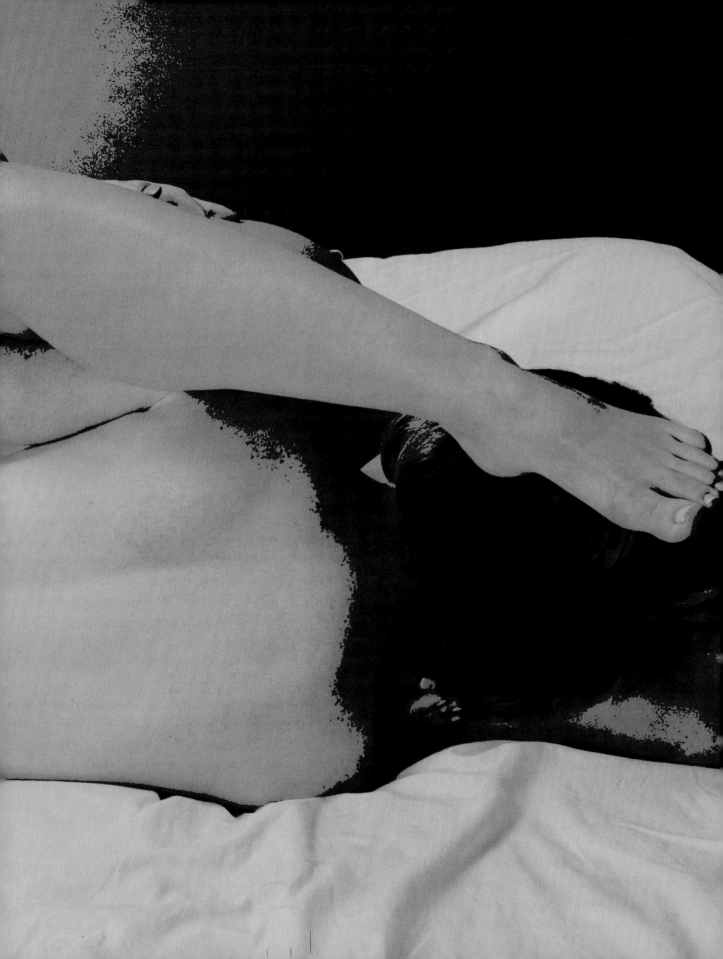

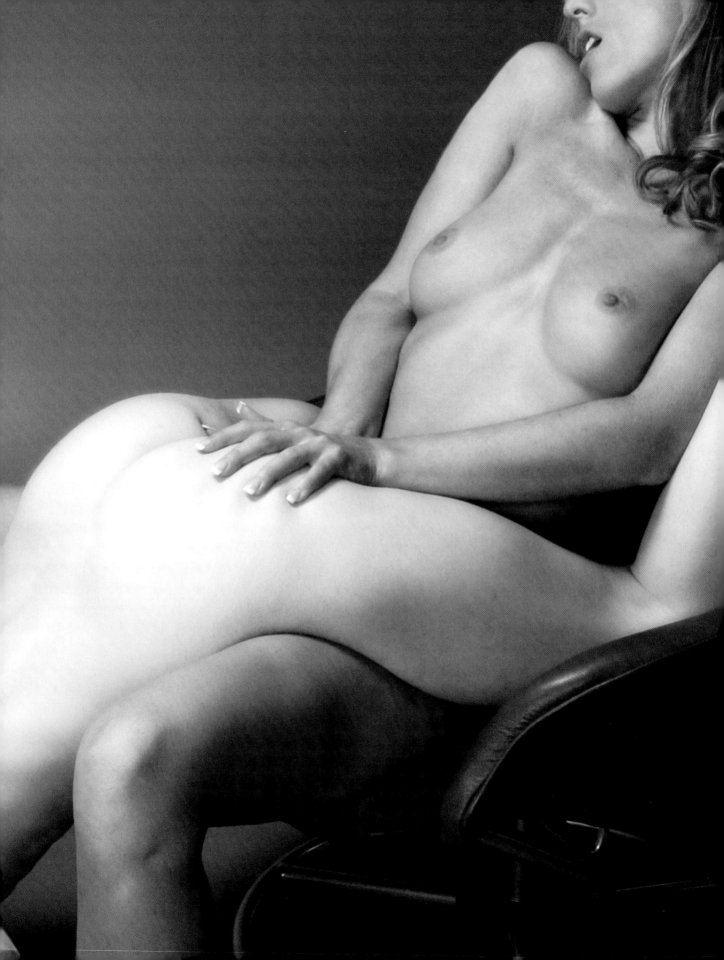

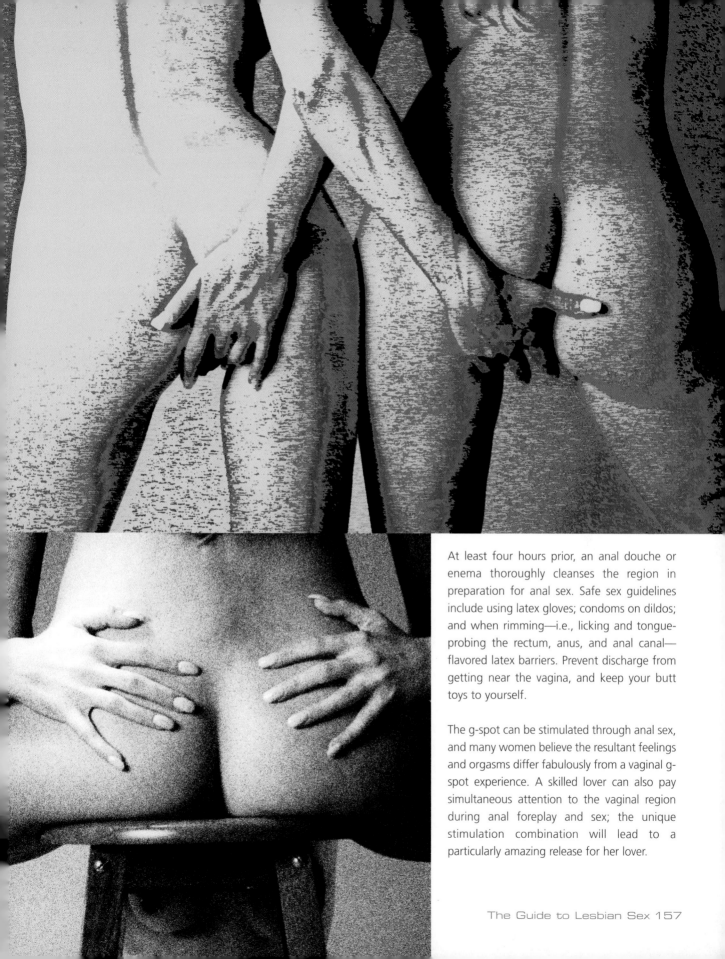

At least four hours prior, an anal douche or enema thoroughly cleanses the region in preparation for anal sex. Safe sex guidelines include using latex gloves; condoms on dildos; and when rimming—i.e., licking and tongue-probing the rectum, anus, and anal canal—flavored latex barriers. Prevent discharge from getting near the vagina, and keep your butt toys to yourself.

The g-spot can be stimulated through anal sex, and many women believe the resultant feelings and orgasms differ fabulously from a vaginal g-spot experience. A skilled lover can also pay simultaneous attention to the vaginal region during anal foreplay and sex; the unique stimulation combination will lead to a particularly amazing release for her lover.

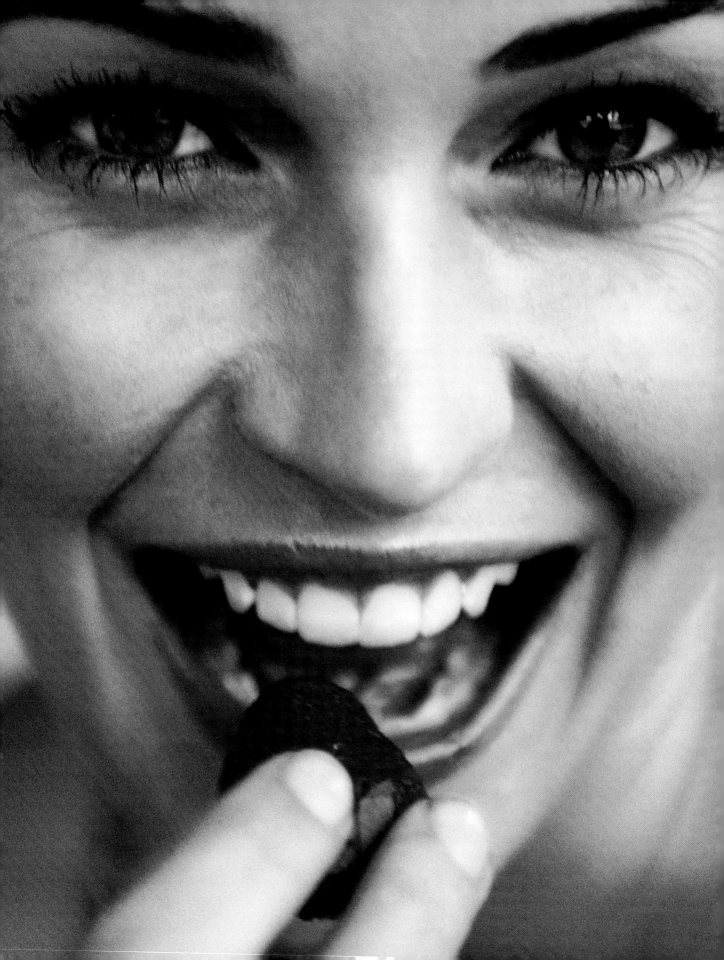

splosh

Erotic food-play is a sensual activity that explores the sexual appeal of condiments and food. Sploshing in the literal sense is the act of making a splashing sound, but to those in the know, sploshing describes one of the most decadent types of food-play fun. Lovers splosh to become sticky, slippery, sloppy, slick, and exceptionally delicious.

The "victim" of the splosh sexcapade tosses her peacock tail to the wind, allowing her lover to dirty her up in order to wipe her down. It's a forbidden thrill beyond the cherished childhood memory of stomping through a mud puddle in one's finest dress clothes.

Prolong the anticipation by first grocery shopping together. You'll look at food displays in a whole new light. Envision the warm, viscous oatmeal being rubbed into your skin by your beautiful lover. Experience the flavor sensation of a fresh peach cobbler commingling with her pussy's natural nectar as you slowly lick it off her inner thighs.

While unpacking the groceries, open the jar and indulge one another in a dip from the honey stick. Cover her with extra virgin olive oil then climb on top and press yourself onto her glistening body.

The splosh may be a gushing and rousing time one night, and a tame, tease, and texture-focused event the next.

Depending on how carried away the splosh session becomes, your messy loving can be carried out on the kitchen floor or even in the bathtub if you are cautious of the slippage factor. Rubber sheets are available through splosh-friendly retailers. It is advised that sploshing be enjoyed on the surface only. Food should not be inserted as it can cause all sorts of infections. Depending on the menu and, mood, foods and condiments can be applied with a squeeze bottle, an eye droplet, a paint brush, or even a bucket.

Drip chilled chocolate pudding onto her nipples. Dip a taste with your finger and insert it into her mouth to treat her to a sampling before slurping the rest off her breasts. Pour maple syrup or warm berry sauce down the length of her body and spend extra time licking the sweet extravagance off her backside.

Lather her up with whipped cream for the dual excitement of highly charged application and removal. Crème fraiche can be enjoyed alone or can top squishy gelatin, chocolate syrup, or any other luscious dessert concoction. Whipped cream is additionally recommended as costuming for an impromptu fashion show or a round of foreplay wrestling.

For a creative lover, an after-dinner liqueur need not be served in a mere snifter. Sip a fine port wine from her belly button, then draw on her midriff with the sediment. The next morning, surprise her at the breakfast table by spreading jam on your bare breasts rather than on your bare muffin. This little eye-opener may make you both late for work, but you'll arrive with a smile on your face.

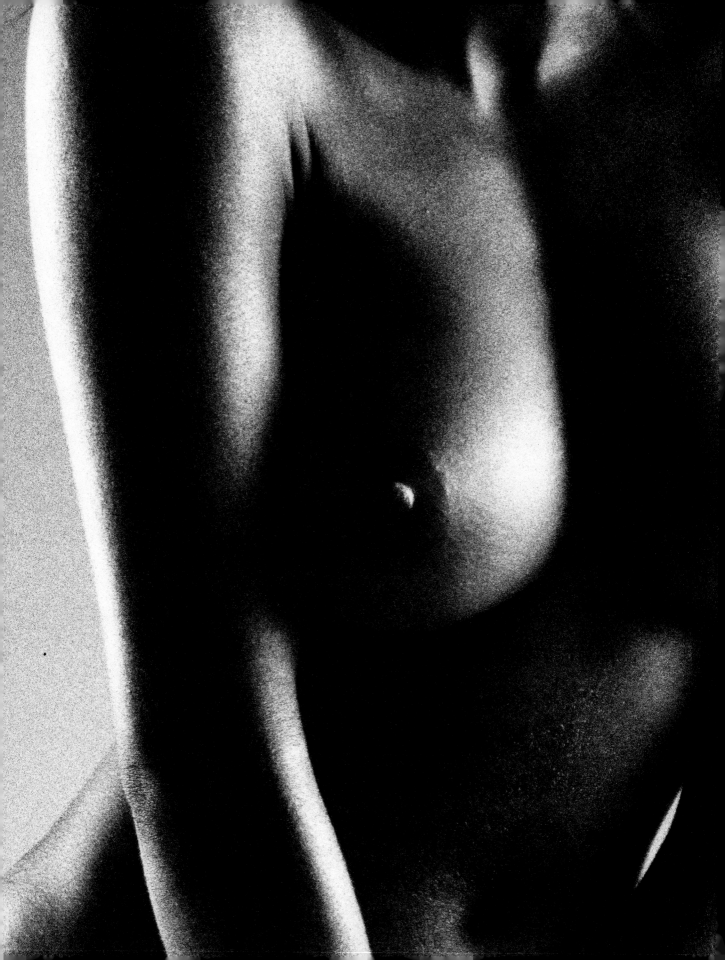

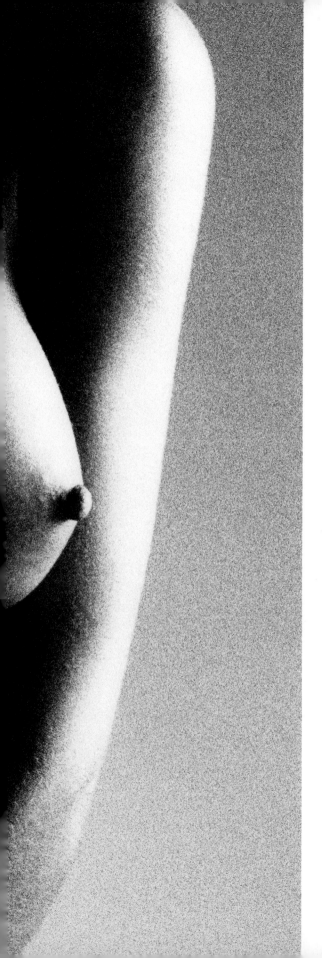

These beautiful glands have been raised to the level of cultural obsession. Most likely because of the heart, the bosom is considered the center of our emotions and feelings, and their milk-producing quality has breasts considered to be revered as a symbol of fertility.

breasts

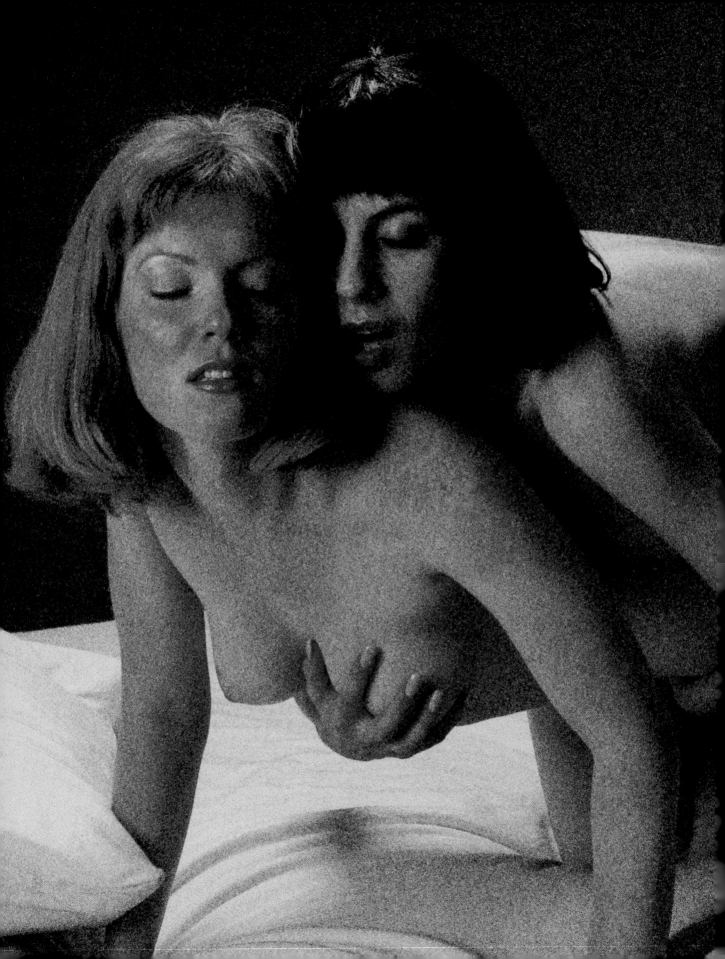

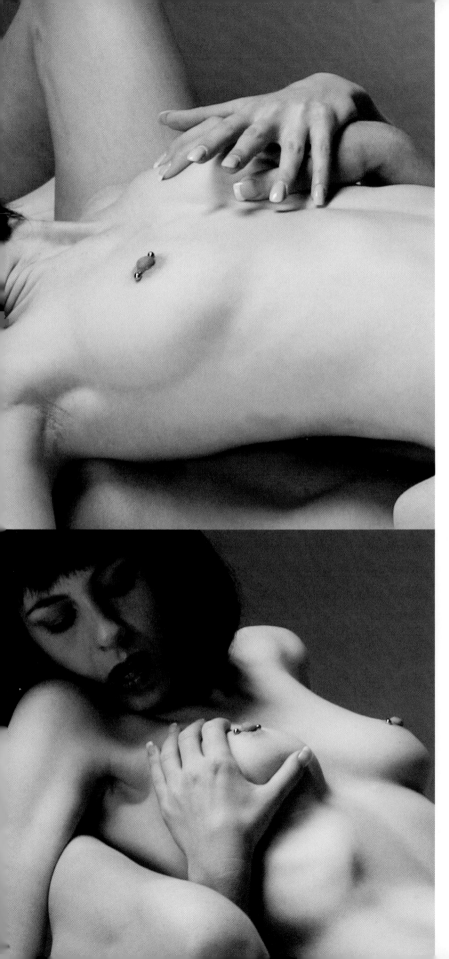

Breasts represent consummate female sexuality. They differ greatly in size, shape, areola color, and sensitivity. We have been encouraged to admire and envy full, matching breasts best exhibited by perfect posture, a beauty standard that is difficult to attain. Even the most confident and beautiful woman needs your reinforcement. Communicate to her how much you love to indulge in her unique bosom. Whether perky, voluptuous, or small, women are acutely aware of this part of their body and the many implications of the powers associated with them—tits and cleavage as a lure, as it were.

The bosom is a superb erotic region. Caress your own breasts the next time you are fiddling around downtown. Choreograph some techniques on yourself before performing them on her. By cupping, fondling, and tracing with your fingers her breasts and nipples during foreplay, her body adjusts to your touch and kisses prior to any move down to her nether regions.

Breasts, whether real or cosmetically enhanced, tend to be most sensitive on the surface, so although especially large breasts seem to beg for more aggressive handling, begin with a gentle, soft caress and work your way to the nipple. If she's into breast play, her nipple will harden. An unanticipated squeeze can make for an exciting jolt as the foreplay heats up.

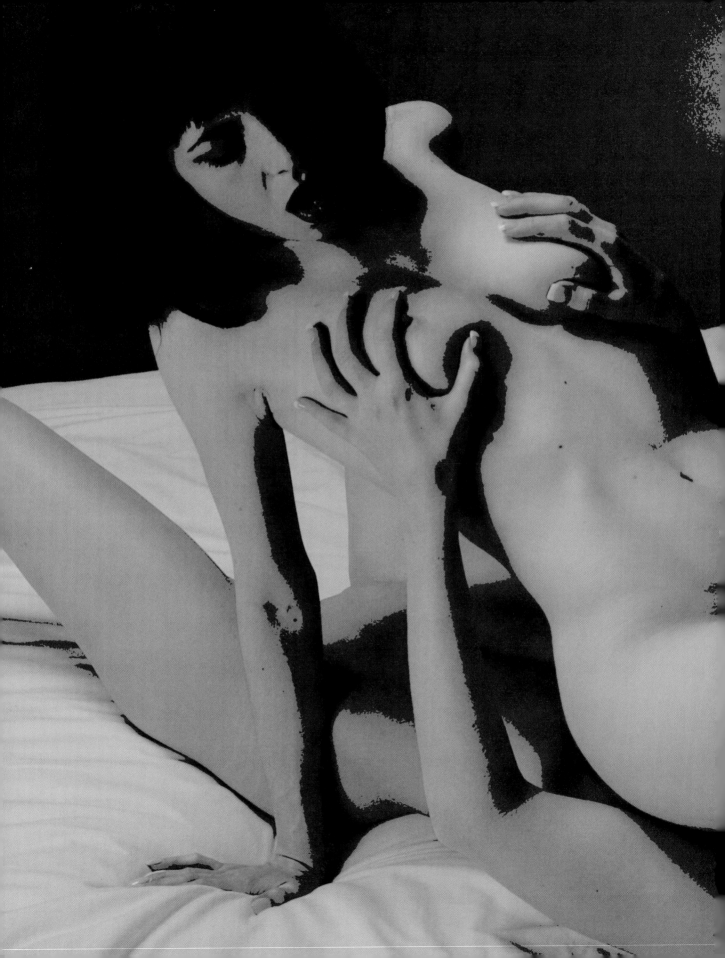

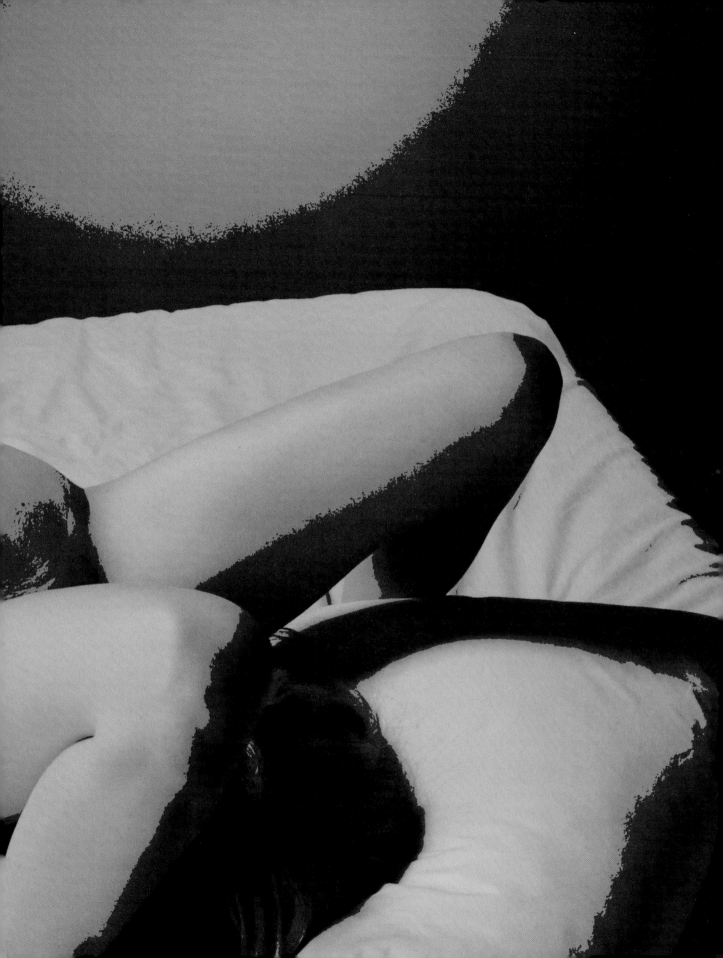

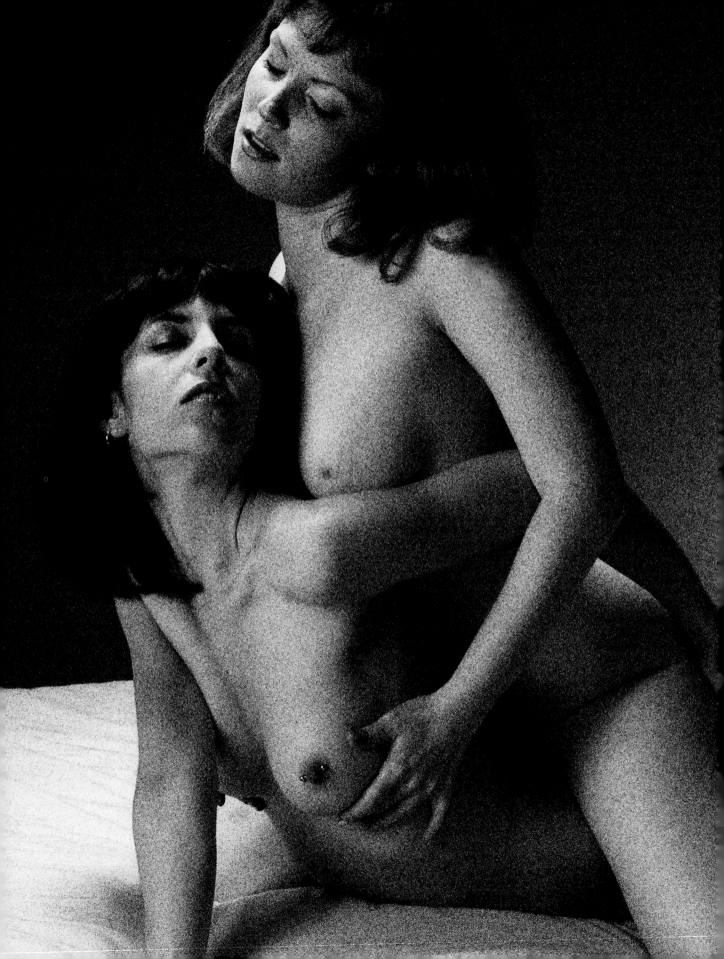

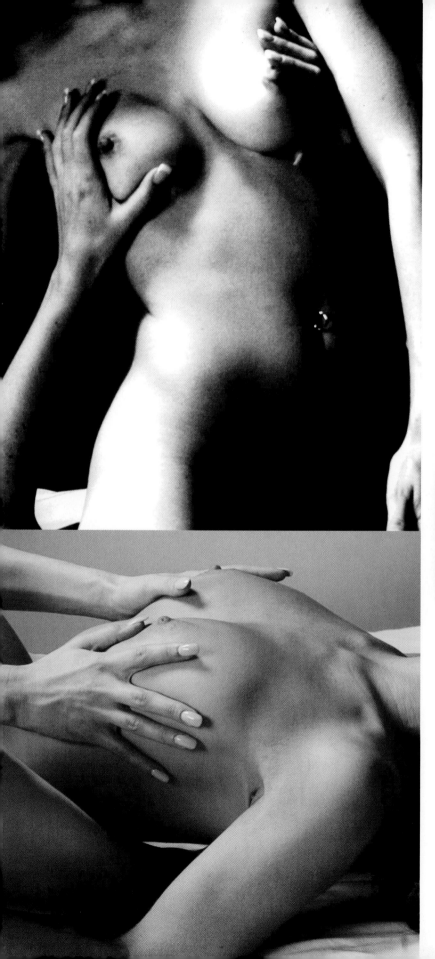

Nipples can also be suckled and tugged. You can use nipple clamps, clothespins, or barrettes. If her nipples are pierced, little bells attached to the breasts make for an unusual and celebratory lovemaking session. These breast props also allow and encourage hands and the mouth to venture to other areas of the now hyper-sensitive body.

During lovemaking, be creative and remember to return to the breasts, as they are much more than a foreplay arena. Use vaginal juices to moisten her nipples as you reach up to caress a breast while simultaneously going down on her, a sexy move known as the "Cherry Picker." Play with your own breasts or nipples during sex. She can't be everywhere at once. A huge turn-on for both partners is to rub your breast onto other areas of her luscious body. For the highly recommended "Nip, tuck," technique, cup your breast and press it into her aroused, moist pussy.

She took my hand and rubbed it over her breast. I felt her nipples become pronounced through her cotton tee and was compelled to feel her erect nipples on the entire map of my hand; gently from the tips down the length of my fingers, against the outer edges of my hand and back into the center of my palm. She watched me and smiled, then helped me remove her shirt.

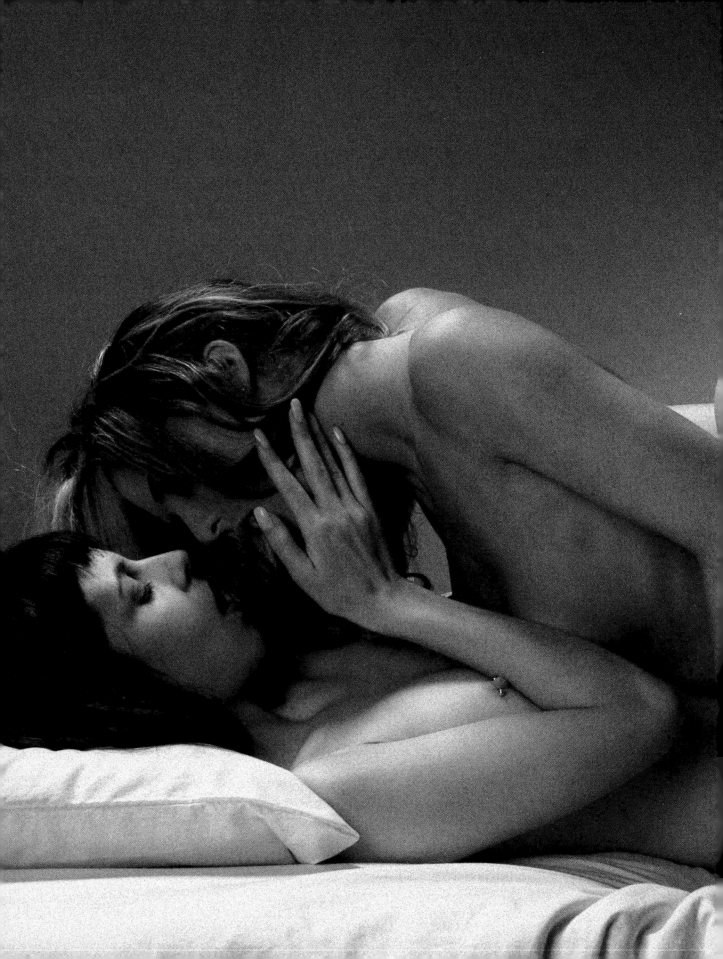

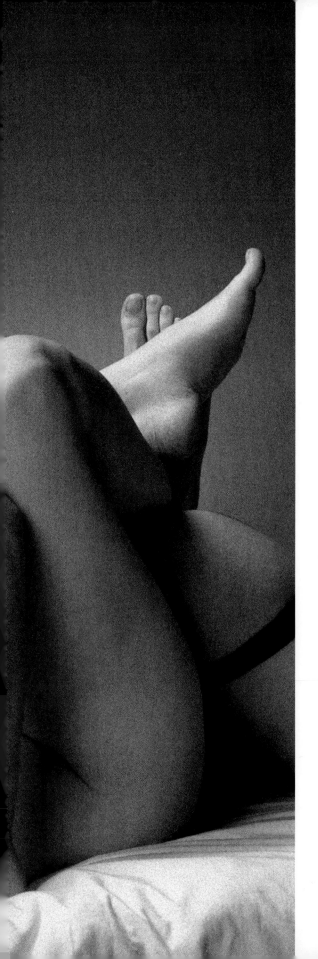

Yes, lesbians do fuck. They fuck well and long and hard and happily and everything in between. *Fuck* is a remarkable word, deployed resoundingly and effortlessly worldwide as a noun, verb, adjective, expletive, and adverb, or to express astonishment, desire, anger, deception, and to highlight or expound upon everything in between.

fuck

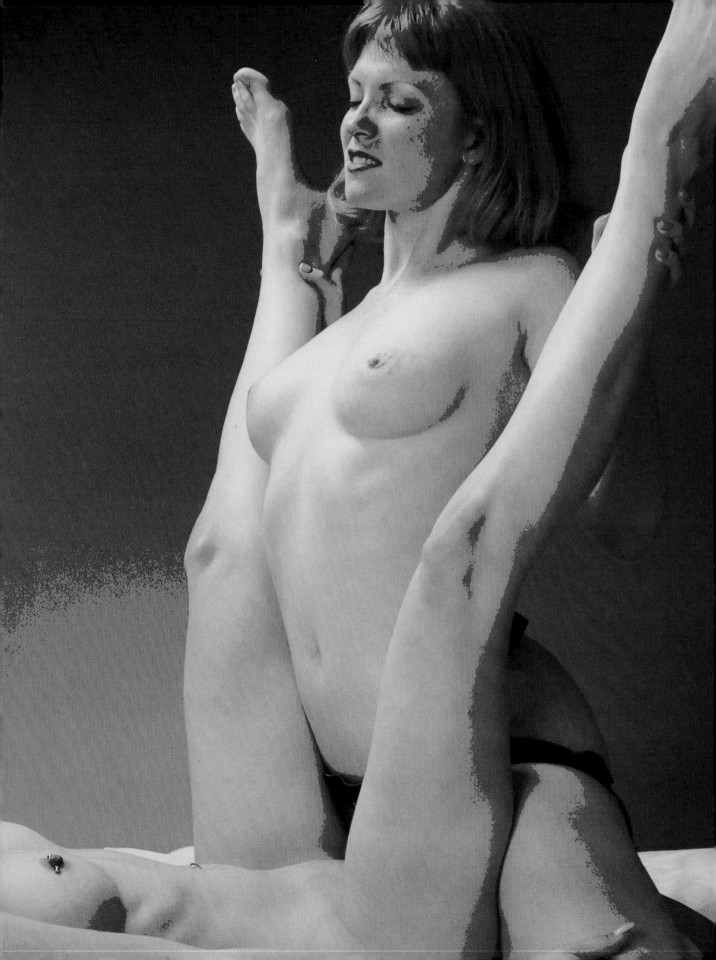

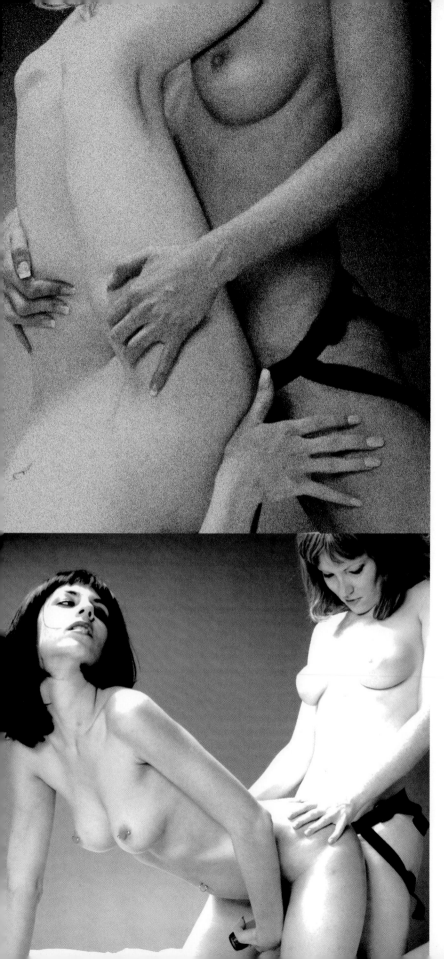

The word *fuck* has been around for at least 500 years, but much disagreement exists as to the etymology of the word. It could be derived from the German, Latin, or Middle English. The urban legend acronyms "for unlawful carnal knowledge," supposedly posted above the stockades of the punished, or "fornication under consent of the king," posted above approved brothels, are overwhelmingly agreed to be historical poppycock. As far as evolved meaning, fuck may have been considered an acceptable word through the 18th century in some cultures before being judged profane and forever doomed to combating censorship. Fuck is among the most well-known, translated, used, and controversial words in the world.

Fuck generally means to be penetrated in some way, as in sexual intercourse. And as much as lesbians enjoy the many activities of "outercourse," most get off on some form of intercourse too. There are many lovemaking acts, but there's something about fucking that is the ultimate in shared experience, bodies humping in a sexy, glorious rhythm, tingling, glistening, flexing, swaying, and pulsating together.

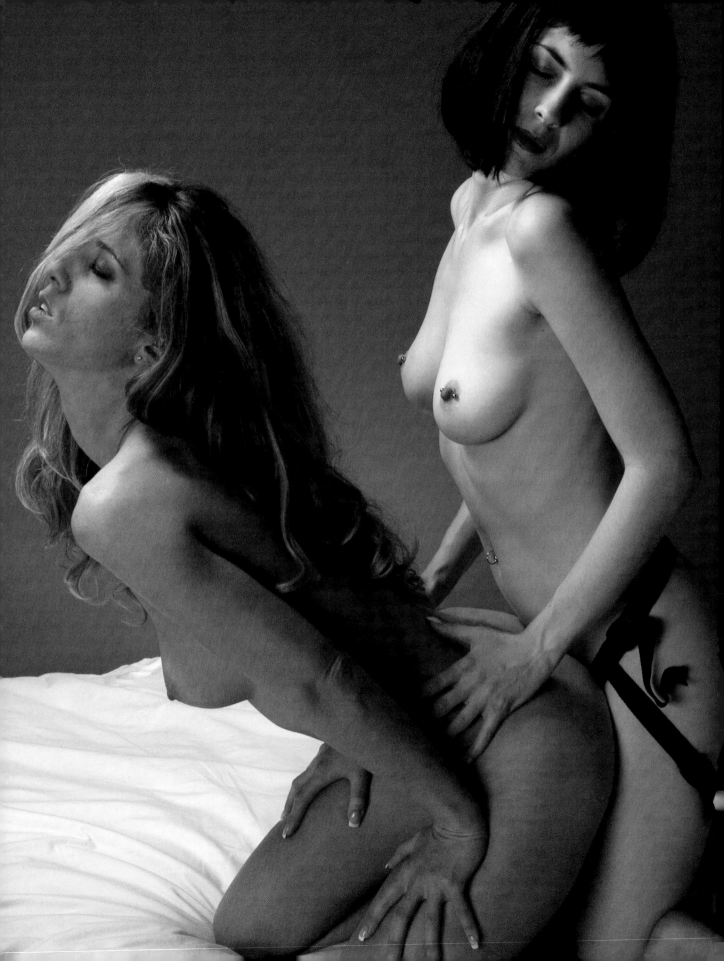

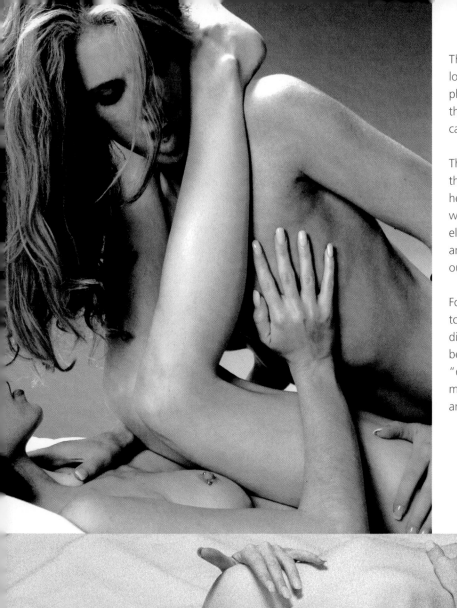

The thrill of entering your lover during lovemaking is exhilarating emotionally and physically. To allow her lover inside is one of the deepest most intimate comforts a woman can bestow another.

Then there's power. It feels extraordinary to thrust into your lover, aggressively showing her, over and over and over, how much you want to please her to the point of quivering elation. Look into her eyes as you enter her and begin to find the rhythm, thrusting in and out of her until you are both satisfied.

For sex, lesbians use primarily their hands, tongues, and lips, supplemented by vibrators, dildos, and other toys. The great thing about being a chick is you can choose the size of the "dick." Keep an assortment for different moods, positions, and types of sex, whether anal, oral, or vaginal.

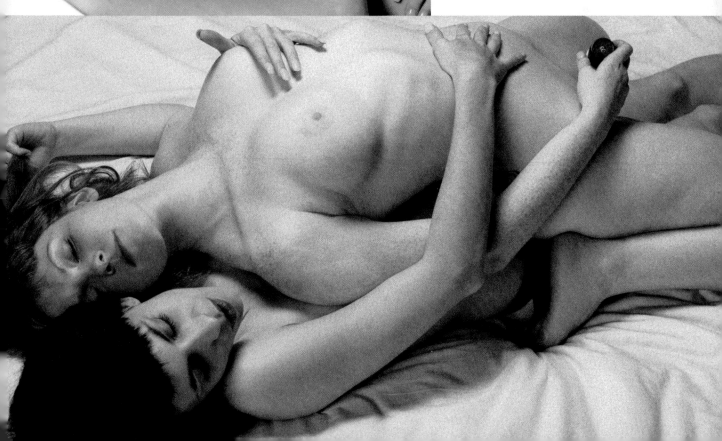

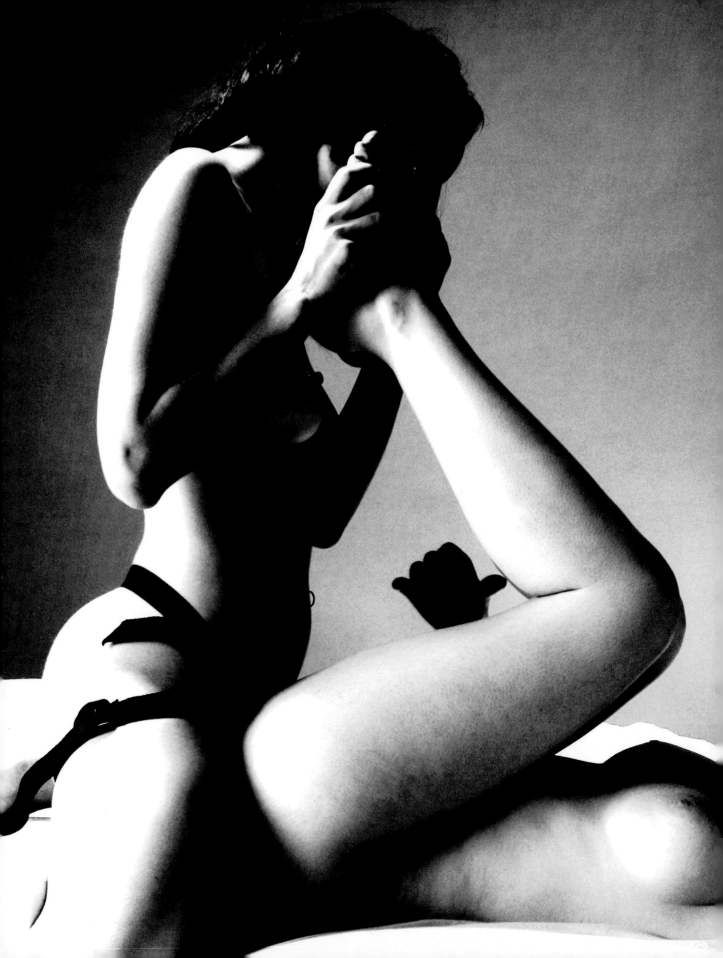

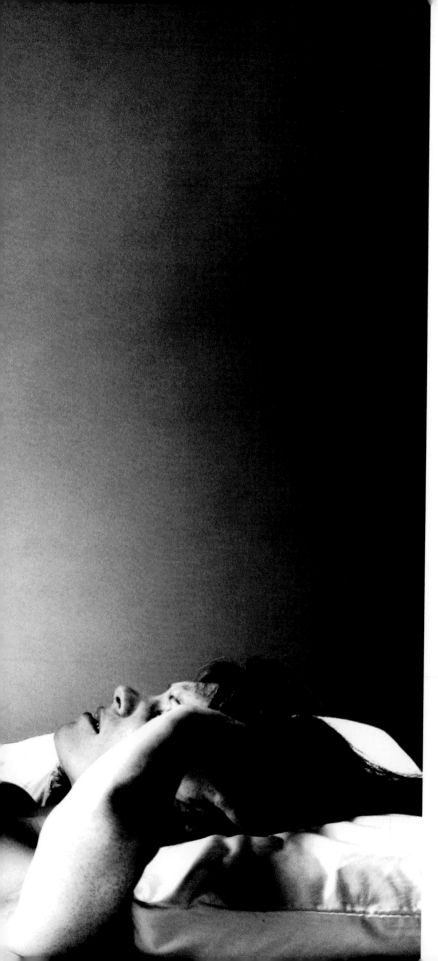

Different positions will stimulate us in unique ways. Here's a sampling:

Vanilla: For this traditional missionary position, legs are open and either flat or with knees tucked to the chest. Slight variations such as one leg extending, draping over a shoulder, or both legs wrapping around your lover are encouraged.

Best in Show: The receptive partner is on all fours allowing her partner to fuck her from behind.

On the Side: Sideways sex, again, entering her from behind.

On Top: Straddling or squatting over your lover allows the top to choose the speed and depth of penetration. During sex, the top can also grind so that her clit rubs against her lover.

Standing: Do it against a wall with one leg raised for easier access.

Saturn's Rings: Women can fuck each other simultaneously. Lovers are seated, facing one another in a near embrace, pussies scooted forward, legs bent and intertwined. The women thrust their pelvises forward and back so that the fingers of their lover enter in and then out of the vagina. If using a double dildo, lubricate, insert into both vaginas, hold the sex toy firmly as needed until the humping rhythm takes over, then swivel pelvises together in an elliptical motion.

Great sex is all about finding the best fit between lovers. It also helps to be healthy and limber, but mastering different positions and becoming an expert lover requires only a willingness to try, humor while learning, and practice. Skill makes love unending.

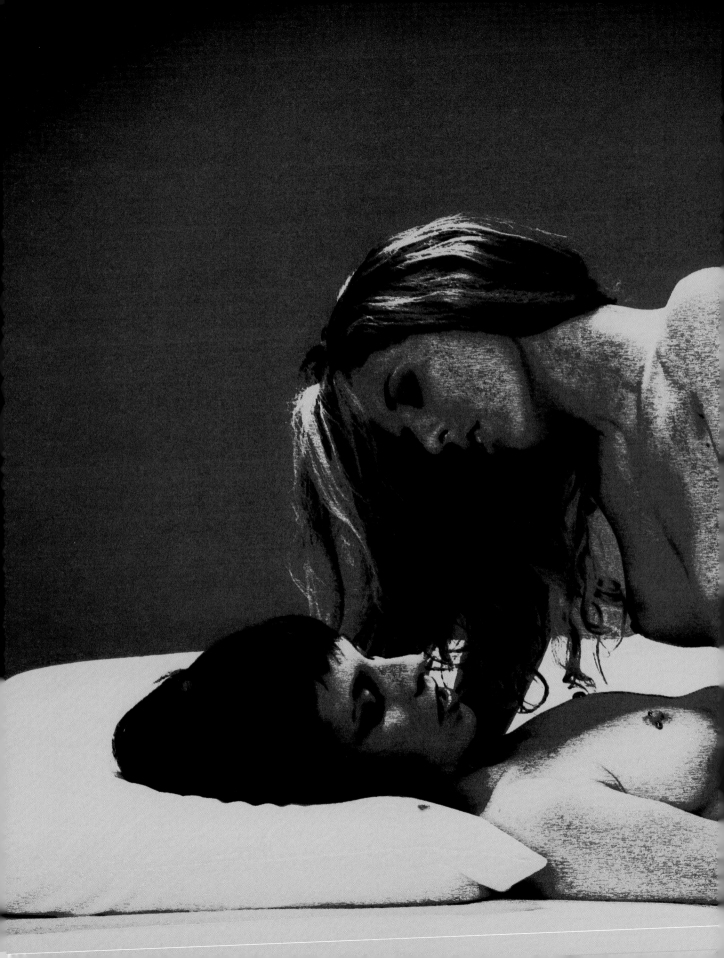

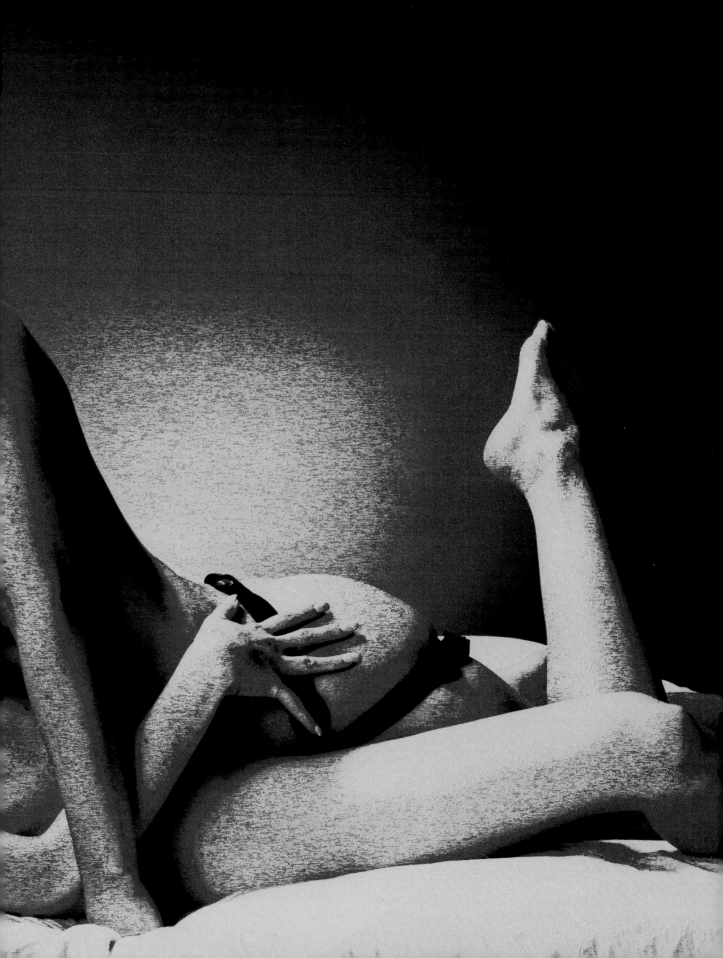

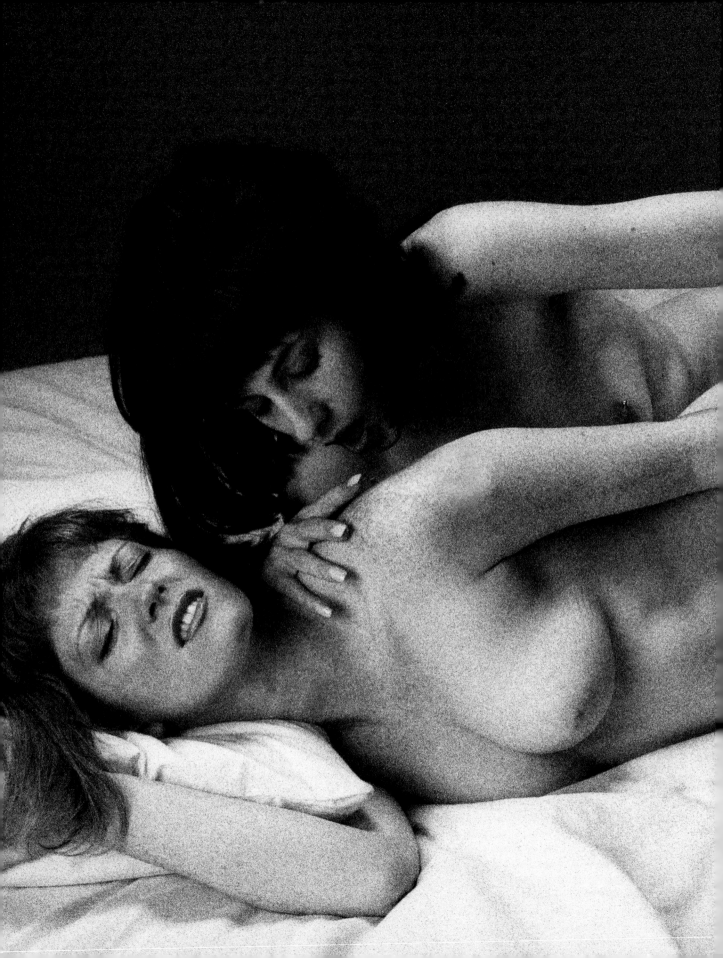

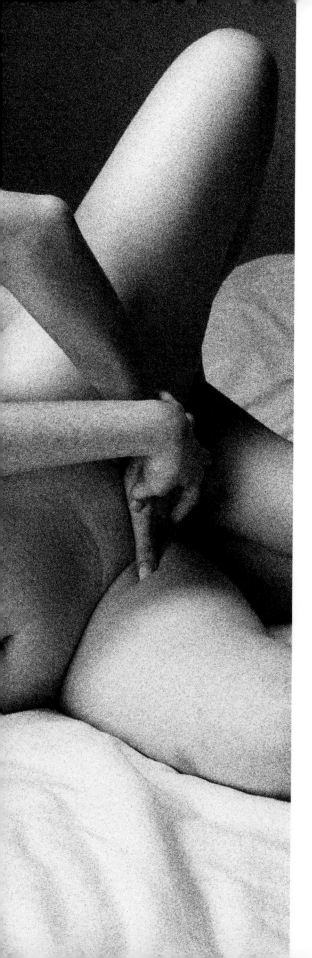

The pièce de résistance of sexual excitement for women is usually characterized by intense pleasure and endorphin rushes, involuntary, rhythmic contractions in the vagina, rectum and/or uterus, and for some, ejaculation. With each sexual activity, orgasmic contractions vary in intensity, duration, and expanse of the body. Achieving a climax is different for each woman each time. Women have the ability to feel different types of climaxes and can experience orgasms involving the vagina, clitoris, rectum, and g-spot. A combination of penetration and direct, constant clitoral stimulation often leads her to the grand finale.

climax

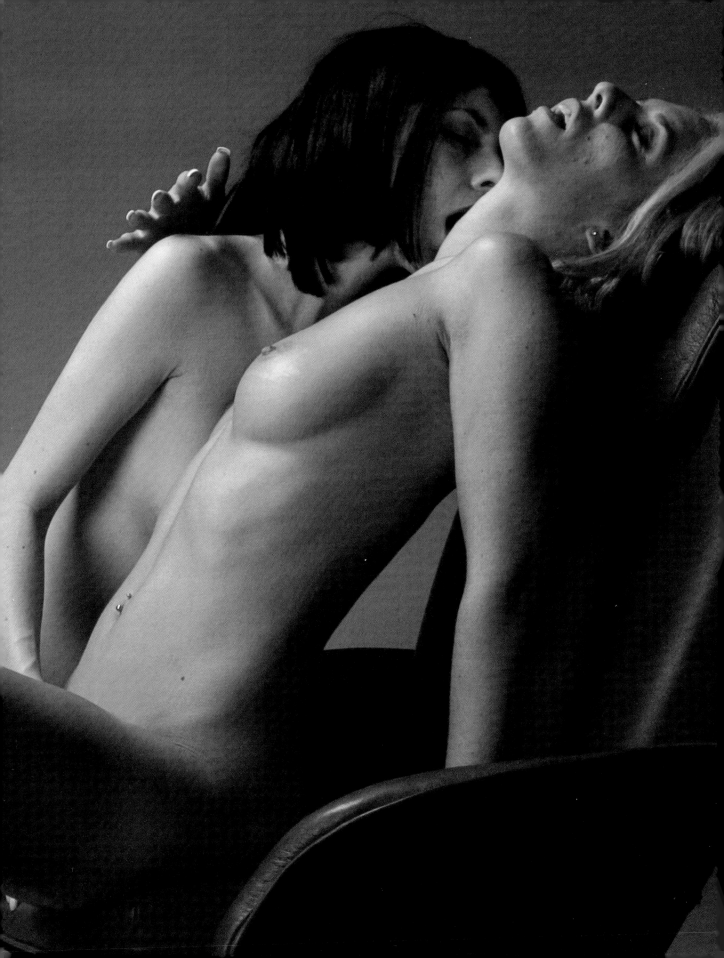

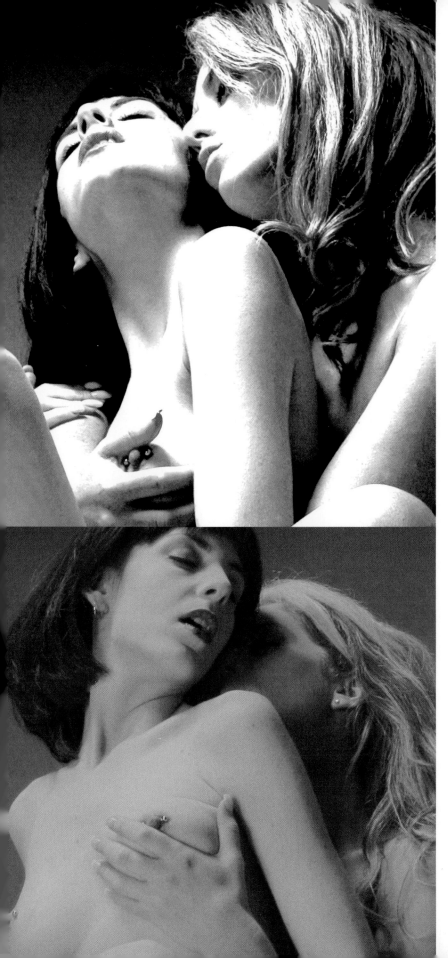

Over the ages, as women have expanded their sexual horizons, their primary sex organ, the clitoris, has also evolved, growing longer, larger, and more sensitive to accommodate our demand for sexual gratification. There are upwards of 8,000 nerve fibers in the crown of the clit, the most dense nerve supply of any part of our skin, and thus a major pleasure zone.

The g-spot, located on the anterior of the vaginal wall, about one-third of the way up, surrounds the urethra and enlarges when aroused, ultimately leading to the release of a unique fluid or ejaculate into the urethra, which some women in turn expel. It may be a drip for some and a gush for others, and skilled women can actually shoot their ejaculate, a completely unique chemical composition, for many feet. Generally, ejaculation occurs when her g-spot is stimulated, but female ejaculation is not always linked to the g-spot or accompanied by an orgasm.

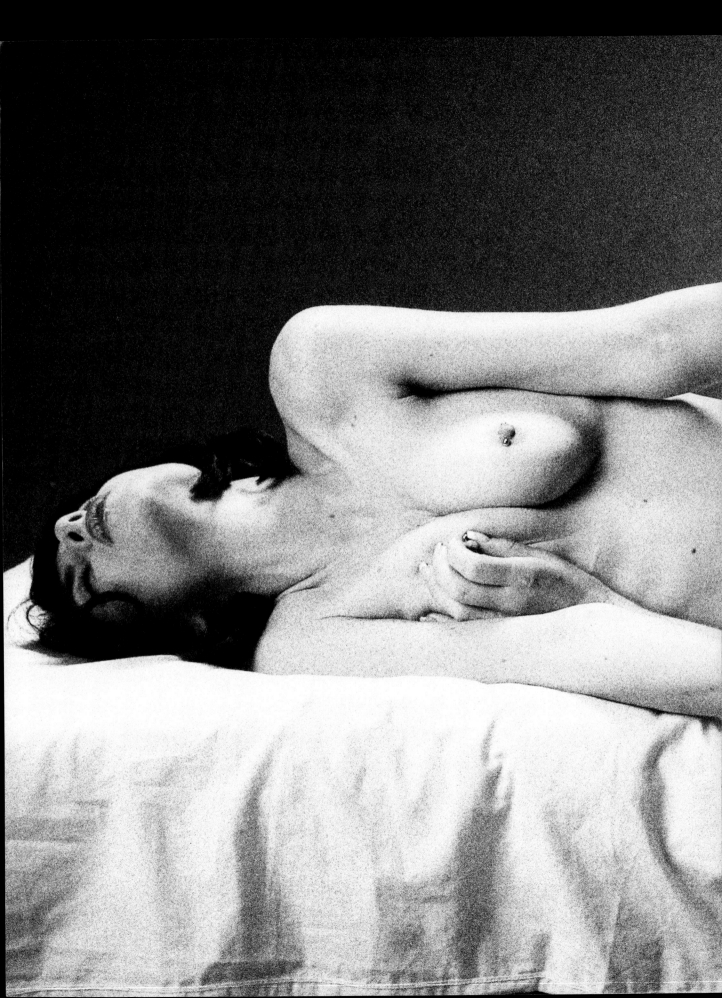

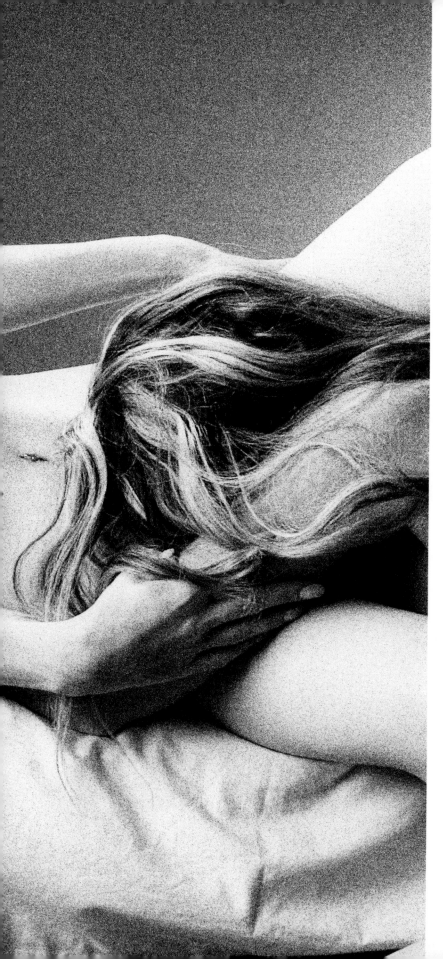

The wall between the anus and vagina is thin, so the g-spot can also be stimulated from an anal entry point. The ideal position or angle varies with each partner, but the consensus is that to stimulate the g-spot, firm pressure is a must. Rhythmically press up into the vaginal ceiling then pull downward in a stroking movement to set in motion the powers of this magic button.

In addition to being able to stay excited for a prolonged period of time after climaxing, for women, recovery time between climaxes is minimal or nonexistent. She may be swollen and sensitive, but can usually continue to make love if all the continuing attention is not placed directly on the tip of her clitoris. Not all women enjoy the same degrees of stimulation, and what feels wonderful for one woman may be uncomfortable or even painful for another.

Although genital stimulation is the most common path to climax, some women can orgasm from prolonged touching of their nipples, for example. Much of our ability to climax resides in our minds.

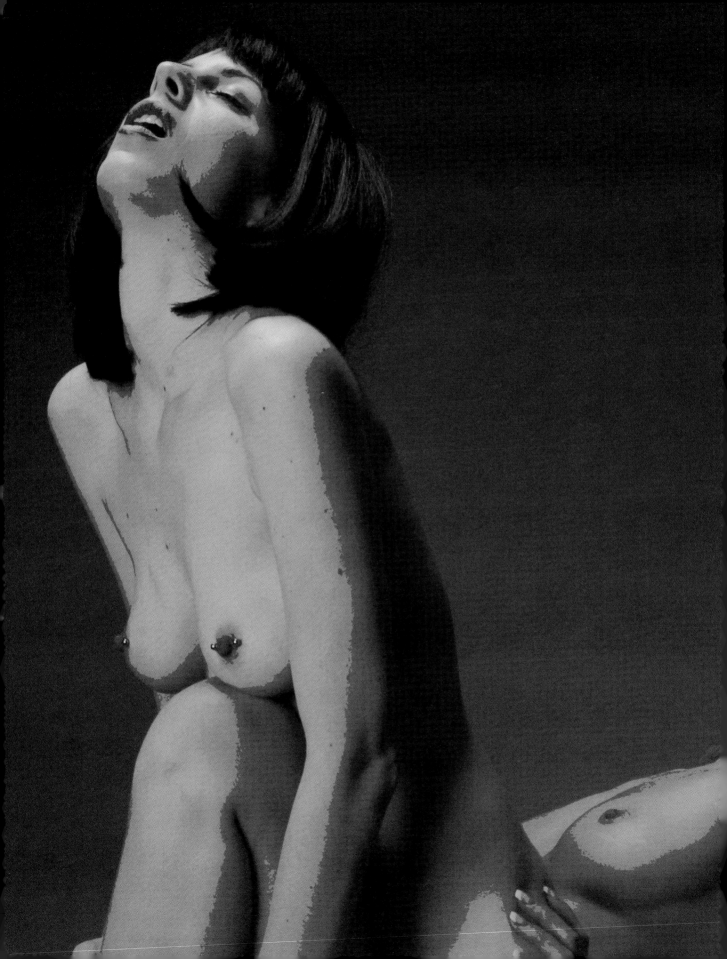

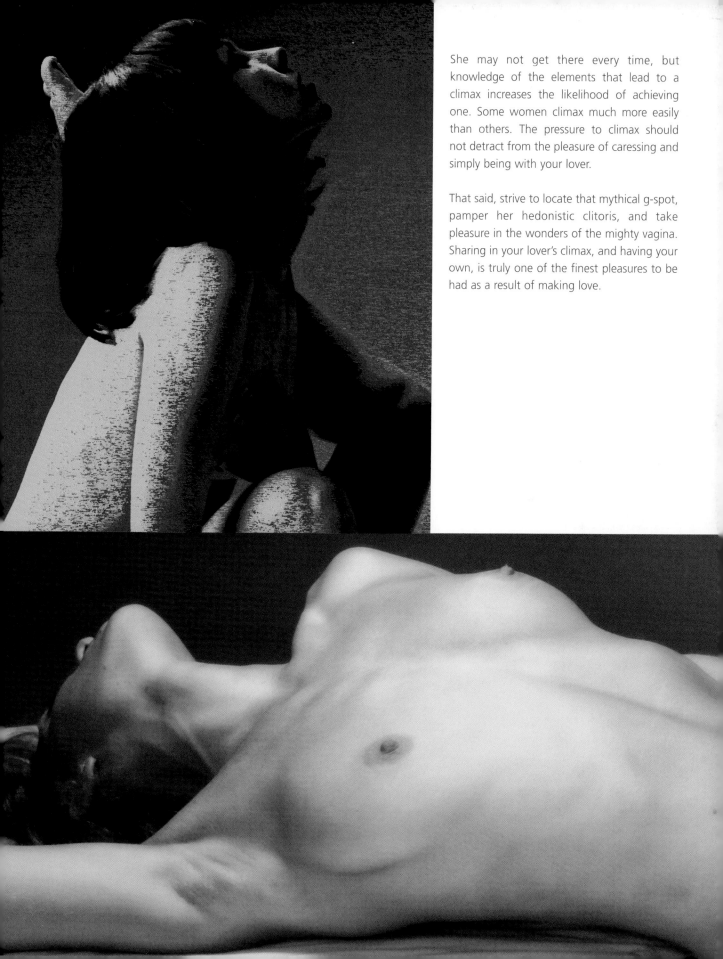

She may not get there every time, but knowledge of the elements that lead to a climax increases the likelihood of achieving one. Some women climax much more easily than others. The pressure to climax should not detract from the pleasure of caressing and simply being with your lover.

That said, strive to locate that mythical g-spot, pamper her hedonistic clitoris, and take pleasure in the wonders of the mighty vagina. Sharing in your lover's climax, and having your own, is truly one of the finest pleasures to be had as a result of making love.

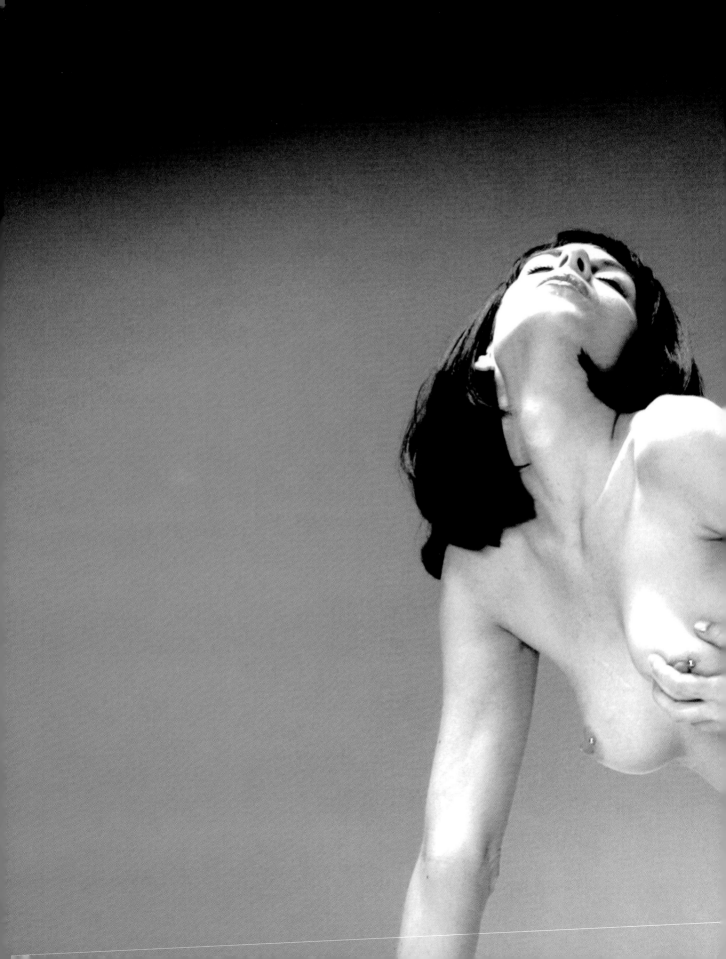

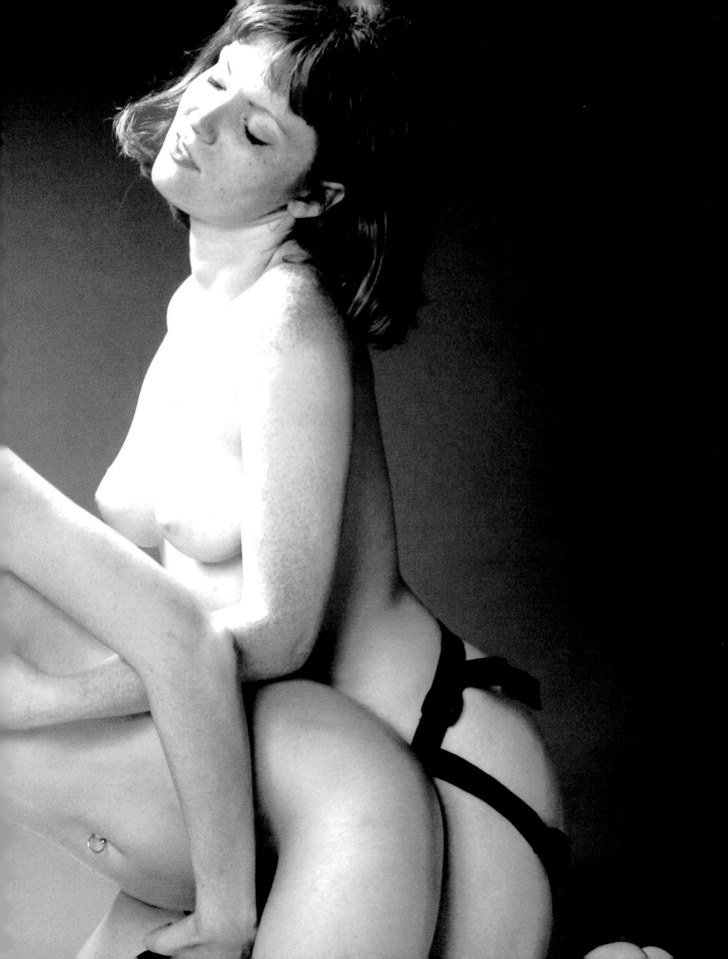

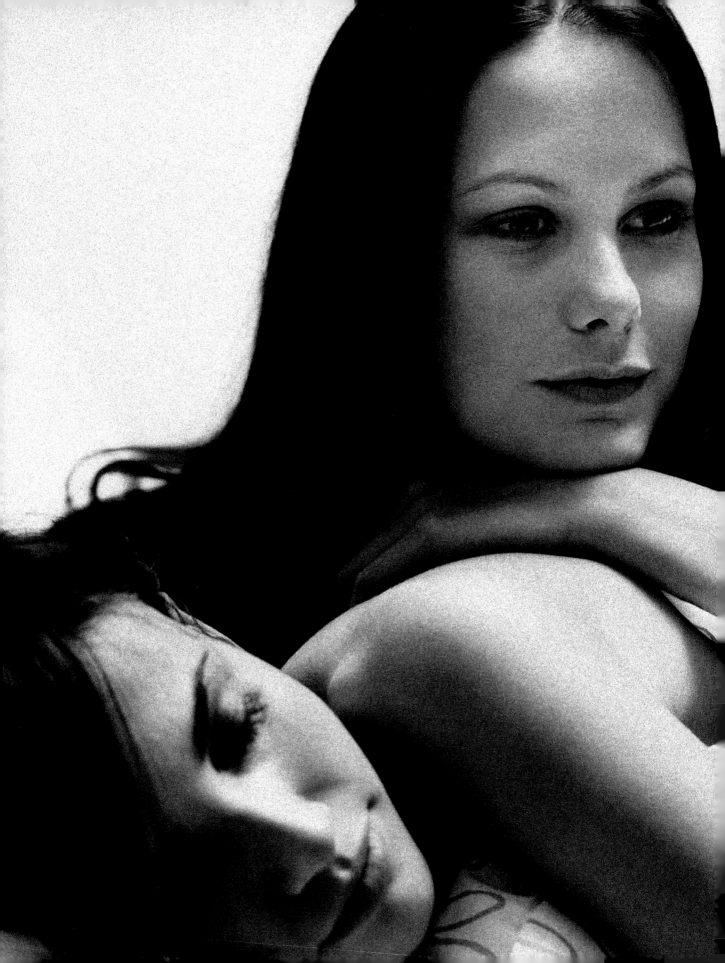

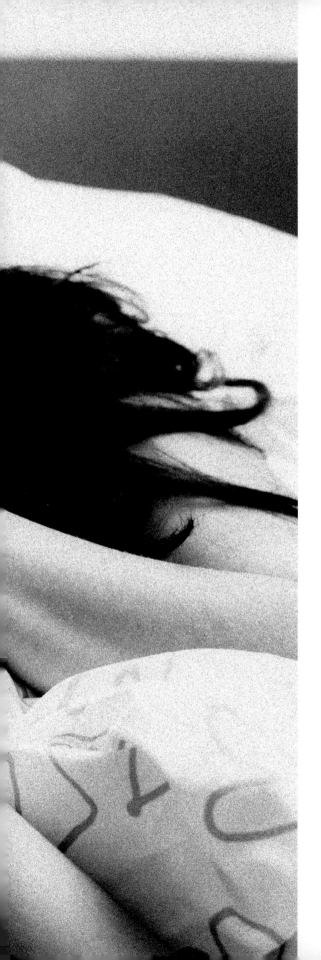

appendix

Appendix

Maintain a healthy sex life. Play safe and be clean, honest, and consensual in every sexual activity. Seek out proper, professional treatment including gynecological and general medical care, and emotional counseling for any health concern you may have, especially regarding sexually transmitted diseases.

There are many reliable internet, retail, and academic sources available. Take responsibility to seek out the information and utilize the resources that are readily available to you.

Bibliography

Annie Sprinkle: Post-Porn Modernist, Annie Sprinkle (Cleis Press, 1998).

The Clitoral Truth: The Secret World at Your Fingertips, Rebecca Chalker (Seven Stories Press, 2000).

Exhibitionism for the Shy, Carol Queen (Down There Press, 1995).

Femalia, edited by Joani Blank (Down There Press,1993).

Good Vibrations: The New Complete Guide to Vibrators, Joani Blank and Ann Whidden.

A Guided Tour of the Collected Works of C.G. Jung, Robert H. Hopcke (Random House, 1989).

The Hite Report: A Nationwide Study of Female Sexuality, Shere Hite (Dell, 1976).

My Secret Garden: Women's Sexual Fantasies, Nancy Friday (Pocket, 1998).

On Our Backs Guide to Lesbian Sex, edited by Diana Cage (Alyson Books, 2004).

Our Bodies, Ourselves for the New Century, The Boston Women's Health Collective (Touchstone, 1999).

"Plump Up the Volume," Vicky Koren (*Daytona Beach News-Journal*, Oct. 11 2005).

The Psychology of Kundalini Yoga: Notes of the Seminar Given in 1932, Carl Gustav Jung, edited by Sonu Shamdasani (Princeton University Press, 1999)

Re-Making Love: The Feminization of Sex, Barbara Ehrenreich, Elizabeth Hess and Gloria Jacobs (Anchor, 1986).

Sex for One: The Joy of Selfloving, Betty Dodson (Crown, 1996).

Sex Toys 101: A Playfully Uninhibited Guide, Rachel Venning & Claire Cavanah (Fireside 2003).

Sexual Behavior of the Human Female, Alfred Charles Kinsey (WB Saunders, 1953, reprinted 1998)

Skin: Talking About Sex, Class & Literature, Dorothy Allison (Firebrand Books, 1994).

Susie Bright's Sexual Reality: A Virtual Sex World Reader, Susie Bright (Cleis Press, 1992).

Three Essays on the Theory of Sexuality, Sigmund Freud (1905).

The Ultimate Guide to Anal Sex for Women, Tristan Taormino (Cleis Press, 1997).

The Whole Lesbian Sex Book, Felice Newman (Cleis Press, 1999).

Why We Love: The Nature and Chemistry of Romantic Love, Helen Fisher (Henry Holt, 2004).

Select Resources

The Advocate
Babeland.com
Bettydodson.com
Bitch
Bomb
Bondage.com
Bust
Curves
Diva
Gatesofheck.com
Gayhealth.com
Gir(L)
Girlfriends
Go NYC
Goodvibes.com
Grandopening.com
HX
Lesbians on the Loose
Lespress
Libidomag.com
Nerve.com
On Our Backs
Out Magazine
Paper
PlanetOut.com
Puckerup.com
Sexuality.org
She
TimeOut

Acknowledgments

Special thanks to my editor extraordinaire, Gail Greiner, and to Sean Moore, Karen Prince, Gus Yoo, Marian Purcell, and all the other sparkling talents at Hylas Publishing. Thanks, too, to David Schmerler, Bonnie, Bob, and Berta, everyone at Babeland, my smart and sexy friends and colleagues, and the sex educators and feminists who continue to educate, intrigue, and inspire me, helping to provide the knowledge and confidence to write and offer up to all of you *The Guide to Lesbian Sex.*

About the Author

Previous to writing about female sexuality, Jude Schell has been an art dealer, a bartender in a lesbian piano bar, and has been involved in film and theater production and publicity. Jude divides her time between Manhattan and Miami. This is her first book.